# Clinician's Manual:
# Treatment of Hypertension

**Third Edition**

**Franz H Messerli**
Director, Hypertension Program
St Luke's-Roosevelt Hospital Center
1000 Tenth Avenue
New York, NY

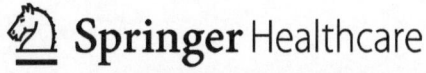

Published by Springer Healthcare Ltd, 236 Gray's Inn Road, London, WC1X 8HB, UK

www.springerhealthcare.com

©2011 Springer Healthcare, a part of Springer Science+Business Media

British Library Cataloguing-in-Publication Data.

A catalogue record for this book is available from the British Library.

ISBN 978-1-907673-08-5

Project editor: Nadine Lemmens
Designer: Joe Harvey
Production: Marina Maher

# Contents

# Author biography

**Franz H Messerli, MD, FACC, FACP,** is Director of the Hypertension Program, Division of Cardiology at St Luke's-Roosevelt Hospital and Professor of Clinical Medicine at Columbia University, College of Physicians and Surgeons in New York City, NY, USA.

Dr Messerli received his MD degree from the University of Bern Medical School, Switzerland. He completed his internship and residency at the Department of Medicine, University Medical School in Bern, Switzerland. Dr Messerli completed a fellowship in cardiology at University Medical School in Bern, Switzerland, and carried out a hypertension cardiology research fellowship at the Clinical Research Institute in Montreal, Canada.

Dr Messerli is the author and co-author of more than 700 publications and book chapters. He has served on the Cardiorenal Advisory Committee of the US Food & Drug Administration (FDA) and Joint National Committee. He is a member of several editorial boards, and has received various awards and degrees for his scientific activity. He is also a Founding Member of the American Society of Hypertension; an Honorary Member of the Southern African Hypertension Society; and an Honorary Fellow or Member of the Philippine College of Physicians, the Brazilian Society of Cardiology, the Bulgarian Society of Cardiology, the Peruvian Society of Cardiology, and the Columbian Society of Cardiology.

# Abbreviations

| | |
|---|---|
| ACCOMPLISH | Avoiding Cardiovascular events through Combination therapy in Patients Living with Systolic Hypertension |
| ACCORD-BP | Action to Control Cardiovascular Risk in Diabetes Blood Pressure |
| ACE | angiotensin-converting enzyme |
| ADA | American Diabetes Association |
| ALLHAT | Antihypertensive and Lipid-Lowering Treatment to Prevent Heart Attack Trial |
| ALPINE | Antihypertensive Treatment and Lipid Profile in a North of Sweden Efficacy Evaluation |
| ALTITUDE | Aliskiren Trial in Type 2 Diabetes Using Cardio-Renal Endpoints |
| ARB | angiotensin receptor blockers |
| ASCOT | Anglo-Scandinavian Cardiac Outcomes Trial |
| BP | blood pressure |
| CALM | Candesartan and Lisinopril Microalbuminuria |
| CHARM | Candesartan in Heart Failure Assessment of Reduction in Mortality and Morbidity |
| CHF | congestive heart failure |
| CI | confidence interval |
| COMET | Carvedilol or Metoprolol European Trial |
| CONSENSUS | Cooperative North Scandinavian Enalapril Survival Study |
| CV | cardiovascular |
| DASH | Dietary Approaches to Stop Hypertension |
| DHP | dihydropyridine |
| EBM | evidence-based medicine |
| FDA | US Food & Drug Administration |
| GFR | glomerular filtration rate |
| HCTZ | hydrochlorothiazide |
| INVEST | International Verapamil–Trandolapril Study |
| JNC | Joint National Committee on Prevention, Detection, Evaluation, and Treatment of High Blood Pressure |
| LDL | low-density lipoprotein |
| LOGIC | Lotrel: Gauging Improved Control |
| LVH | left ventricular hypertrophy |
| MI | myocardial infarction |
| MRC | UK Medical Research Council |
| NSAID | nonsteroidal anti-inflammatory drugs |

| | |
|---|---|
| ONTARGET | ONgoing Telmisartan Alone and in combination with Ramipril Global Endpoint Trial |
| OR | odds ratio |
| RALES | Randomized Aldactone Evaluation Study |
| RAS | renin–angiotensin–aldosterone system |
| SHEP | Systolic Hypertension in the Elderly |
| TNT | Treatment to New Targets |
| Val-HeFT | Valsartan Heart Failure Trial |
| VALUE | Valsartan Antihypertensive Long-term Use Evaluation |

# Chapter 1

# Definition of hypertension

A survey of the literature of the past few decades shows that the definition of hypertension has changed drastically, and it seems to continue to change. It is presently recommended that antihypertensive therapy is started in patients who have "confirmed" hypertension, defined by the Seventh Report of the Joint National Committee on Prevention, Detection, Evaluation, and Treatment of High Blood Pressure (JNC 7) as a blood pressure (BP) level exceeding 140/90 mmHg. However, data from the Framingham Heart Study [1] make it exceedingly clear that BP is directly related to cardiovascular events, even at levels below that defined as hypertensive by the JNC 7 [2]. High normal BP was associated with a several-fold increase of cardiovascular disease in the Framingham population (Figure 1). A number of recent studies have shown that lowering BP in the so-called normotensive population reduces morbidity and mortality. These recent data indicate that any arbitrary definition of hypertension, such as BP of above 140/90 mmHg, may not be very useful. It seems time to abandon the dichotomous partition of the world population into either hypertensive or normotensive.

Target BP should be lower in certain groups of patients (as acknowledged by the JNC 7), such as those with diabetes, renal failure, or heart failure. The recent Action to Control Cardiovascular Risk in Diabetes Blood Pressure (ACCORD-BP) trial has proven this concept wrong: in patients with type 2 diabetes, targeting a systolic blood pressure below 120 mmHg, as compared with less than 140 mmHg, did not reduce total or nonfatal cardiovascular events [3].

- Hypertension may best be defined as "a BP level that increases the cardiovascular risk for a given patient."
- Normotension, or the absence of hypertension, may be defined as "a BP level that has no impact on this cardiovascular risk."
- Hypotension may be defined as "a BP that causes orthostatic symptoms or leads to impairment of blood flow to target organs."

There are, of course, potential pitfalls to such pathophysiologic definitions of hypertension and hypotension. It is entirely conceivable that in some patients BP cannot be lowered to levels that would abolish all cardiovascular and renal risk before the patient experiences distinct orthostatic symptoms or repercussions from decreased blood flow to target organs, resulting in myocardial and/or renal ischemia.

**Cumulative incidence of cardiovascular events in patients without hypertension**

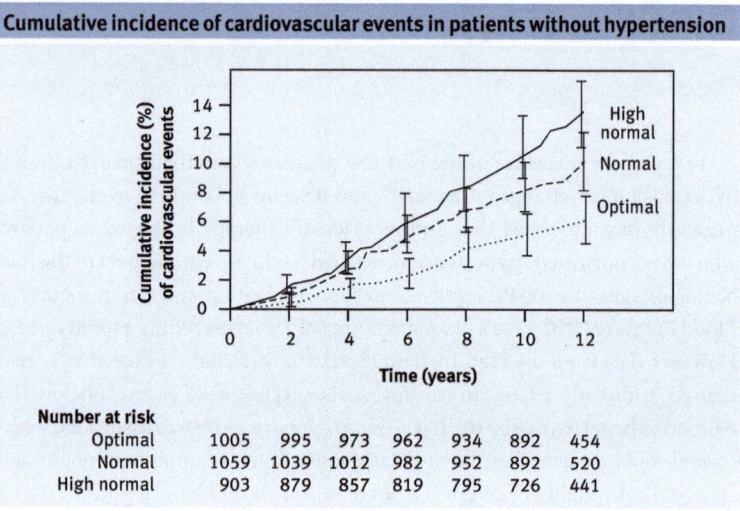

**Figure 1 Cumulative incidence of cardiovascular events in patients without hypertension.** The Framingham data suggest that even within the normotensive range patients with the highest blood pressure (high normal) have a risk of cardiovascular morbidity and mortality that is several times higher than that of patients who have optimal blood pressure. Data from male patients is shown here. Reproduced from Vasan et al. [1].

# Chapter 2

## The J curve

Much ink has been expended on whether the relationship between BP and cardiovascular morbidity and mortality follows a J-shaped pattern. Conceivably, as BP is lowered, morbidity and mortality diminish, but, clearly, there is a point at which further lowering leads to the under-perfusion of vital organs and, thereby, will increase morbidity and mortality. Thus, it stands to reason that a J curve has to exist. However, it is not so clear whether the nadir of the J curve is anywhere near the target range of the systolic or diastolic pressure. Most studies have shown that for both cerebrovascular and renal disease there seems to be no J-shaped curve with regard to systolic or diastolic pressure. However, numerous studies have shown that the issue is different for diastolic pressure and coronary artery disease. The myocardium is perfused almost exclusively during diastole and, therefore, diastolic pressure is critically important for coronary perfusion. Most studies that have examined the relationship between diastolic pressure and the risk of coronary heart disease documented a J-shaped relationship in the physiologic range; namely, diastolic pressures below 85–80 mmHg. In the 22,000-patient International Verapamil–Trandolapril Study (INVEST), a clear J-shaped relationship was found between diastolic pressure and coronary artery disease, but not with stroke or systolic pressure [4]. In this study, all patients had coronary artery disease and hypertension. When diastolic pressure was below 70 mmHg, the risk of myocardial infarction (MI) doubled; when diastolic levels were below 60 mmHg, the risk quadrupled.

More recently, a distinct J-curve relationship between BP and primary outcome was found in the 15,000-patient Valsartan Antihypertensive Long-term Use Evaluation (VALUE) study [5], the 10,000-patient Treatment to New Targets (TNT) trial [6], and in the 25,000-patient ONgoing Telmisartan Alone and in combination with Ramipril Global Endpoint Trial (ONTARGET) trial [7]. In some of these trials, the J-curve relationship between systolic and diastolic pressure and the primary outcome remained unchanged after propensity matching, indicating that a low BP portents an increased risk of future cardiovascular events.

In general, BP lowering is still not tackled aggressively enough, and only about a third of all patients with hypertension are controlled according to the JNC 7 criteria [8]. However, in patients at risk, such as those with manifest coronary artery disease, excessive lowering of diastolic pressure could have serious consequences. In contrast, it can be assumed that, as long as there is significant proteinuria in a patient with diabetes, arterial pressure is inappropriately elevated to levels that are detrimental for the kidney. This could lead to the paradoxical situation whereby one target organ, such as the kidney, requires a BP that the other target organ, the heart, cannot afford. Thus, many questions remain as to the exact target level for BP during antihypertensive therapy in a given patient. The good news, however, is that lowering BP to values below 140/90 mmHg has been shown to drastically reduce cardiovascular morbidity and mortality, and to be safe in the large majority of patients with hypertension. Importantly, the majority of patients with uncomplicated hypertension will need two or more drugs to lower BP levels to meet therapeutic goals.

# Chapter 3

# Drug therapy or lifestyle modification?

The lifestyle modifications recommended by the JNC 7 were mostly nutritional, consisting of weight loss in the overweight, lowering of dietary sodium intake to less than 100 mmol/day, modification of alcohol intake to, at most, two drinks per day, and maintenance of an adequate dietary intake of potassium, calcium, and magnesium [2]. The JNC 7 also recommended regular physical activity for all patients with hypertension who have no conditions that would make exercise contraindicated.

There is little doubt that many lifestyle factors, such as dietary salt, alcohol intake, lack of exercise, and stress, can affect BP and contribute to hypertension. Conversely, it has been well documented that BP can be lowered by modifying lifestyle. The antihypertensive efficacy of lifestyle modification in four thorough meta-analyses of a large number of patients has been reported [8–11]. Although the fall in BP may appear relatively small, it should not be forgotten that, in contrast to drug therapy, lifestyle modification has few, if any, adverse effects and may also exert a favorable effect on concomitant risk factors, such as hyperlipidemia, insulin resistance, obesity, and gout (Figure 2). Implementing lifestyle modifications, as effective as they are, is often very difficult and discouraging, and physicians have learned that repeated nagging about weight loss, a low-salt diet, and regular exercise may adversely affect the physician–patient relationship.

My recommendation is that, once the diagnosis of hypertension has been established, the patient should be treated with pharmacologic therapy. This by no means indicates that lifestyle modifications have no place in the anti-hypertensive approach. As soon as the BP is under control (and this rarely takes longer than a few weeks), ample time remains to educate the patient with regard to dietary modifications, weight control, and exercise. In fact, any exercise prescription is much less risky in a patient whose BP is well controlled than in a patient who has uncontrolled hypertension (ie, has an elevated baseline BP and an exaggerated BP response during peak exercise). Patients soon realize that it is much more convenient to pop a pill than to try to follow restrictive dietary recommendations for the rest of their lives.

Many patients are unwilling, or unable, to live up to the high expectations of lifestyle modification. Also, there seems little reason to expose the vascular tree of a patient, and its target organs, to an elevated pressure for months before antihypertensive therapy is started. Importantly, there is no justification to deny antihypertensive therapy to patients who are unable to modify their alcohol intake to the desired two drinks a day, to overweight patients who are unable to shed the necessary pounds, or to smokers who are unable, or unwilling, to give up cigarettes. To the contrary, BP needs to be aggressively treated in such patients because they have comorbid factors that greatly accelerate the long-term repercussions of hypertensive cardiovascular disease.

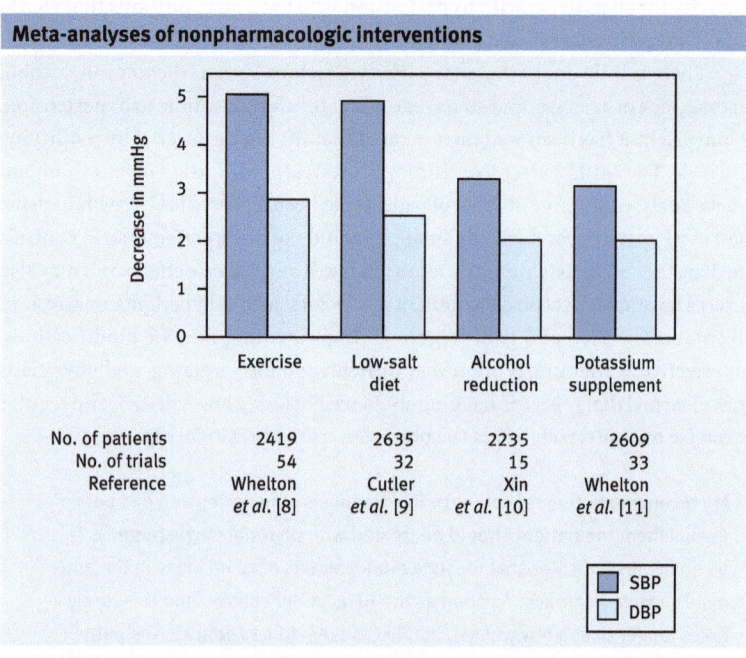

**Meta-analyses of nonpharmacologic interventions**

| | Exercise | Low-salt diet | Alcohol reduction | Potassium supplement |
|---|---|---|---|---|
| No. of patients | 2419 | 2635 | 2235 | 2609 |
| No. of trials | 54 | 32 | 15 | 33 |
| Reference | Whelton *et al.* [8] | Cutler *et al.* [9] | Xin *et al.* [10] | Whelton *et al.* [11] |

Figure 2 **Meta-analyses of nonpharmacologic interventions.** DBP, diastolic blood pressure; SBP, systolic blood pressure.

## Low-salt diet

Lifestyle modifications can profoundly affect antihypertensive therapy; for instance, a low sodium diet will decrease potassium excretion in a patient who is on a diuretic, as less sodium is available at the level of the distal tubule for exchange against potassium. Thus, a low-sodium diet will prevent total body potassium depletion and, thereby, may enhance the morbidity and mortality benefits of diuretic therapy. In the Systolic Hypertension in the Elderly (SHEP) study [12], patients who had hypokalemia showed no reduction in heart attacks and strokes when compared with patients whose potassium was normal, despite a similar fall in BP. In addition, by stimulating the renin–angiotensin–aldosterone system (RAS), a low-sodium diet also enhances the antihypertensive efficacy of angiotensin-converting enzyme (ACE) inhibitors and angiotensin receptor blockers (ARBs). Not only is BP lowered more efficiently with ACE inhibitors and ARBs in a patient on a low-sodium diet, but also the beneficial effects of these drugs on proteinuria (and the progression of renal disease) are distinctly enhanced. As shown in the Dietary Approaches to Stop Hypertension (DASH) trial [13], a diet that emphasizes fruit and vegetables will lower BP, even when patients do not restrict their salt intake, although the combination of such a diet with sodium restriction had the greatest antihypertensive effect.

> My dietary advice to all patients with hypertension is sound and simple, and consists of three parts:
> eat lots of fresh fruits and vegetables;
> avoid processed or prepared food; and
> stay clear of the salt shaker at the table and in the kitchen.

A very high potassium intake has been shown, on occasion, to be detrimental in patients on ACE inhibitors and ARBs. In susceptible patients, the ingestion of large amounts of apple juice or dried fruit can cause hyperkalemia, a decrease in glomerular filtration rate (GFR), and an increase in creatinine.

A guide for patients wishing to adopt a healthy diet is provided in Figure 3 [14].

## Weight loss

Numerous studies have shown that weight loss results in a fall in BP. This fall is particularly prominent in patients on a high-protein diet because of the so-called natriuresis of fasting. In susceptible patients, a high-protein diet may lead to dehydration, orthostatic hypotension and even syncope. This scenario is not uncommon in patients who are on blockers of RAS (ACE inhibitors or ARBs) because the activity of the renal angiotensin system is upregulated by the sodium depletion secondary to the high-protein diet. Thus, patients

Recommended food purchases for one person following a healthful diet containing 2100 kcal and 1500 mg of sodium per day*

| Type of food | Servings per wk | Serving size | Total amount purchased per wk | Recommendations |
|---|---|---|---|---|
| **Weekly purchases** | | | | |
| Market periphery | | | | Do most weekly shopping in this section |
| Vegetables† | | | | |
| Leafy greens | | | | |
| Salad greens | 4 | 1 cup | 1–2 bags or heads | Lettuce, mixed spring greens, spinach bunch (about 1 lb) |
| Other greens | 4 | ½ cup | 1–2 bunches | Kale, collard greens, mustard greens (about 1 lb) |
| Cruciferous | 3 | ½ cup | 1–2 heads | Broccoli, cabbage, cauliflower (about 1 lb) |
| Colorful‡ | 15 | ½ cup | 8–12 individual items | Tomatoes, carrots, squash, peppers, sweet potatoes, corn, eggplant, avocados (about 3 lb) |
| Other | 3 | ½ cup | ½ lb | Celery, green beans, peas, lima beans, sprouts |
| Fruits | | | | |
| Fresh | 20 | 1 medium or ½ cup chopped | 15–20 individual items | Apples, pears, grapes, bananas, peaches, plums, oranges, tangerines, berries, cantaloupe, pineapple |
| Dried | 8 | ¼ cup | 1 bag | Raisins, apricots, prunes, cherries (about ½ lb) |
| Juice | 4 | 1 glass (8oz) | 1 qt | Orange, grapefruit, unsweetened carrot |
| Herbs, alliums, and other seasonings | Use freely | | | Thyme, ginger, garlic, onion, bay leaf, lemon juice |
| Meat, poultry, and fish | | | | |
| Fish and shellfish | 2 | 6–8 oz | 1 lb | Cod, sea bass, halibut; fresh or canned salmon, tuna, or sardines; mollusks, shrimp, crabmeat |
| Poultry | 2 | 6–8oz | 1 lb | Turkey, chicken, low-sodium cold cuts |
| Red meats | 1 | 2–4 oz | ¼ lb | Beef, pork, lamb, low-sodium cold cuts |
| Dairy products | | | | |
| Milk | 10 | 1 glass (8 oz) | ½ gallon | Choose low-fat or nonfat products |
| Yogurt | 3 | 1 cup | 1 container | Choose low-fat or nonfat products (about 32 oz) |
| Cheese | 4 | 1 slice | ¼ lb | Soft or hard |
| Processed-food aisles§ | | | | Choose only low-sodium products¶ |
| Nuts (whole or butter) | 10 | 1 oz | 1 bag or jar | Walnuts, almonds, peanuts (about ½ lb) |

| Item | | | | Examples |
|---|---|---|---|---|
| Legumes | 3 | 1 cup | 1 can or bag | Chickpeas, lentils, black beans (about 1lb) |
| Olives | 2 | 1/2 cup | 1 jar | Black, green, stuffed (about 1/4 lb) |
| Spices | Use freely | | | Black pepper, cayenne, cinnamon, paprika |
| Baked goods | 20 | 1 slice | 1 bag | Bread, rolls, pancakes, waffles (about 1 1/2 lb); choose wholegrain products |
| Tomato products | 4 | 2/3 cup | 2 jars or cans | Sauce, juice, whole or diced (about 12 oz per jar or can) |
| Chips and other snacks | 3 | 1/2 cup | 3 bags | Tortilla chips, popcorn, pretzels (about 1 1/2 oz per bag) |
| Chocolate or sweets | 1 | 1 oz | 1 bar or similar amount | Granola bars, chocolate bars (about 1 oz) |
| Other food aisles (sweetened beverages, candy, cookies) | | | | Skip these aisles |
| **Less frequent purchases*** | | | | |
| Breakfast cereals | 2 | 1/2 cup | 1 1/2 cup | Oats, bran, whole wheat flakes, other whole grains |
| Pasta, rice, and grains | 3 | 1 cup (cooked) | 1/2 cup | Pasta, brown rice, bulgur, quinoa, wheat berries |
| Cooking oils | 12 | 1 tbs | 3/4 cup | Canola, corn, sunflower, olive, soybean |
| Table fats | 16 | 1 tsp | 1/3 cup | Soft, oil-based spreads free of trans fat |
| Salad dressings and mayonnaise | 21 | 1 tsp | 1/2 cup | Choose low-sodium items |
| Sugars | 24 | 1 tsp | 1/2 cup | Table sugar, jelly, honey, maple syrup |
| Desserts | 1 | 1/2 cup | 1/2 cup | Ice cream, sorbet, frozen yogurt, other (4 oz) |
| Eggs | 3 | 1 | 3 | Large eggs |
| Salt | 7 | 1/3 cup | 2 1/3 cup | Salt for cooking or added at the table |

**Figure 3 Recommended food purchases for one person following a healthful diet containing 2100 kcal and 1500 mg of sodium per day.**

* Patients should observe the following general recommendations: don't skip meals, and consume one third of daily calorie intake at breakfast; limit eating out to once weekly and choose meals with a low salt content — just one slice of pizza, a turkey sandwich, or a pasta dish can easily contain 2000 mg of sodium. Examples of conversion from standard to metric measures: 1 oz equals 28 g; 1 teaspoon, 5 g; 1 cup leafy greens, about 75 g.

† Unsalted frozen or canned vegetables can be substituted for fresh vegetables.

‡ Choose at least four different types of vegetables from this category.

§ Also visit the processed-food aisle as needed for other food items in the less frequent purchases category.

¶ Look for lower-sodium, unsalted, or reduced-salt items. Compare brands and choose those with lower sodium content. The total amount of sodium consumed in a week from processed foods or eating out should not exceed 2000 mg.

** Weekly allowances are provided for items that are generally purchased less than once a week. The amounts for weekly intake should be set aside in individual containers to make it easier to keep track of how much is consumed.

Reproduced with permission from Sacks & Campos [14].

well controlled on multiple antihypertensive drugs should be warned not to drastically change their diet, as unexpected adverse effects such as weakness and even syncope can occur.

While there is no question that any weight loss over the short term reduces BP, the long-term effects of weight loss have been disappointing. Sjöström et al. [15] has shown that, 10 years after gastric bypass surgery, BP returns to presurgical levels despite the fact that weight loss was sustained and body weight remained more than 15% lower than before surgery.

## Exercise

Regular aerobic exercise is an excellent tool in the antihypertensive arsenal. The exact mechanism of any exercise-induced fall in BP is probably multi-factorial. It may be related to salt and volume depletion caused by sweating and also to conditioning of the large arteries to accommodate a higher stroke volume, thereby rendering them more compliant. In contrast to aerobic exercise, isometric exercise (weightlifting) has not been shown to have a significant effect on BP.

## Step-down therapy

Should the patient be successful in modifying their lifestyle weeks or months after BP is controlled with antihypertensive therapy, it is reasonable to consider using the "step-down" approach to decrease the dose, or number, of anti-hypertensive drugs taken, or even to stop therapy completely. Lowering BP over the long term by using antihypertensive drugs such as ACE inhibitors, ARBs and calcium antagonists, will reduce vascular hypertrophy and target organ disease and will restore endothelial function. After antihypertensive therapy is stopped in a successfully treated patient, it is often possible for that patient to stay off therapy for months, even years, provided that they maintain reasonable lifestyle modifications and monitor their BP regularly [16]. Again, lifestyle modification should not be considered as a substitute for drug therapy in hypertension, but rather should be complementary to drug therapy.

## Antihypertensive therapy in physically active patients

Lifestyle modifications often have to be adapted to fit a specific antihypertensive therapy and vice versa. Regular aerobic exercise has a mild antihypertensive effect, probably because of low-grade, chronic fluid volume and salt depletion. Thus, aerobic exercise should be encouraged in all patients with hypertension; conversely, drugs that decrease aerobic exercise performance, such as beta-blockers and, to a lesser extent, diuretics, should be avoided in the physically active patient. Fluid and salt depletion associated with diuretic therapy may make the patient more prone to dehydration during prolonged aerobic exercise. Isometric exercise (weightlifting) is relatively contraindicated in patients with hypertension because of the excessive spikes in systolic pressure that have been documented during strenuous weightlifting. Profound hypotension can be observed in patients on ACE inhibitors or ARBs, together with dehydration, such as that which occurs when running or when undertaking other aerobic exercise during the hot summer months. With increasing dehydration, the activity of the RAS becomes increasingly important in maintaining BP within the physiological range; blockade of this system takes away the body's most important defense mechanism. Patients who are prone to orthostatic hypotension, such as elderly patients and patients with diabetes, should be warned about dehydration when starting antihypertensive therapy with an ACE inhibitor or an ARB. Calcium antagonists as a class are well tolerated in patients who exercise regularly and have not been shown to impair exercise tolerance. Nevertheless, good control of BP is mandatory in all patients before embarking on an exercise program.

# Chapter 4

## First-line antihypertensive therapy: the simplistic viewpoint

By definition, all antihypertensive drugs lower BP. Given at appropriate doses, the antihypertensive efficacy is remarkably similar among various drugs. However, outcome data and adverse effects have been shown to differ from one drug class to another.

### Outcome

The drug class best documented to reduce morbidity and mortality in hypertension, when compared with either placebo or active therapy, remains the thiazide diuretics, specifically chlorthalidone. In all diuretic-based trials, other antihypertensive drug classes, such as beta-blockers and antiadrenergics, have been added to titrate BP to target. However, although the addition of these drugs to diuretic therapy adds to the antihypertensive efficacy (and therefore, seemingly has a beneficial effect on the surrogate end point), they have not been shown to enhance the benefit of diuretics on morbidity and mortality (the real end point). Thus, it cannot be concluded that the addition of these drugs is beneficial. Even shakier is the conclusion that these drugs by themselves (when not added to diuretics) will be beneficial. In contrast to chlorthalidone therapy, treating hypertension with beta-blockers, for instance, has not been shown to offer any primary cardioprotective or cerebroprotective effect in the patient with hypertension (Figure 4) [17].

Although numerous studies attest to the efficacy of beta-blockers for secondary cardioprotection, there are no data showing that lowering BP with a beta-blocker reduces the risk of heart attack, stroke, or cardiovascular or all-cause mortality. It makes little sense, therefore, to start a patient with hypertension at risk for coronary artery disease or stroke on a beta-blocker. Conversely, ACE inhibitors have been shown to reduce some cardiac end points more than would be expected from their antihypertensive efficacy alone. Thus, a patient at risk for acute MI is likely to profit much more from lowering BP with an ACE inhibitor than from lowering BP to the same extent with a beta-blocker. Diuretics, calcium antagonists and ARBs have been shown to reduce the risk of stroke better than most other drug classes and should, therefore, be the preferred treatment in patients at risk for cerebrovascular disease.

The statement from the JNC 7 [2] that thiazides are "unsurpassed" in reducing morbidity and mortality is, however, unfortunately deceptive. There is no question that in SHEP [18] and the Antihypertensive and Lipid-Lowering Treatment to Prevent Heart Attack Trial (ALLHAT) [19], chlorthalidone was exceedingly efficacious in reducing heart attacks, stroke and death. Similarly, a reduction in morbidity and mortality has been shown in some trials with indapamide [20,21]. However, the most commonly used thiazide diuretic is hydrochlorothiazide (HCTZ), with more than 130 million prescriptions per year in the US alone. Over 95% of HCTZ is used at a dose of 12–25 mg/day. There are no, repeat no, data available showing that such a dose of HCTZ reduces morbidity and mortality. All studies with HCTZ were performed using a much higher dose. Furthermore, a recent meta-analysis has shown that the antihypertensive efficacy of HCTZ in the dose range of 12.5–25 mg is paltry and significantly inferior to all other antihypertensive drug classes [22]. Thus, because of a lack of outcome data at commonly used doses and suboptimal antihypertensive efficacy, physicians should no longer prescribe HCTZ as initial antihypertensive therapy.

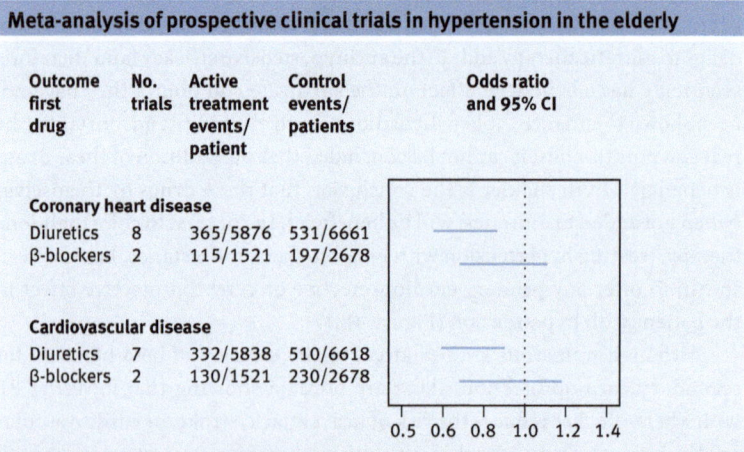

**Meta-analysis of prospective clinical trials in hypertension in the elderly**

| Outcome first drug | No. trials | Active treatment events/ patient | Control events/ patients | Odds ratio and 95% CI |
| --- | --- | --- | --- | --- |
| **Coronary heart disease** | | | | |
| Diuretics | 8 | 365/5876 | 531/6661 | |
| β-blockers | 2 | 115/1521 | 197/2678 | |
| **Cardiovascular disease** | | | | |
| Diuretics | 7 | 332/5838 | 510/6618 | |
| β-blockers | 2 | 130/1521 | 230/2678 | |
| | | | | 0.5  0.6  0.8  1.0  1.2  1.4 |

**Figure 4 Meta-analysis of prospective clinical trials in hypertension in the elderly.** CI, confidence interval. Modified from Messerli et al. [17].

## Adverse effects and tolerability

Most antihypertensive drugs have some adverse effects that can affect tolerability. For instance, the main adverse effect of dihydropyridine calcium antagonists is pedal edema [23], which is dose dependent and more common in women than in men. In an overweight, middle-aged woman, calcium antagonist monotherapy will almost invariably trigger, or aggravate, pedal edema and make the patient unhappy with the selection of the initial antihypertensive drug. Of note, not all dihydropyridine calcium antagonists have an equal effect with regard to pedal edema. For a given fall in BP, lercanidipine, manidipine and lacidipine elicit less edema than do amlodipine and nifedipine.

The great majority of patients with mild hypertension cannot be controlled with monotherapy, but need two or more drugs to lower BP into the target range. Monotherapy rarely lowers BP sufficiently, because it invariably triggers compensatory mechanisms that serve to maintain BP at its "usual pretreatment" level. Treatment with a diuretic, for instance, stimulates the sympathetic nervous system and activates the RAS. The activation of both of these systems will mitigate the antihypertensive efficacy of the diuretic. Thus, it is useful to start therapy with a drug, or a drug class, that can be combined easily or is available as a fixed combination with another drug class. Tolerability may also be an issue in the selection of antihypertensive therapy. The best-tolerated drug class for first-line antihypertensive therapy is the ARBs, followed, on an equal footing, by ACE inhibitors and calcium antagonists, then low-dose diuretics and, finally, considerably less well tolerated, the alpha-blockers and beta-blockers. **From a simplistic, tolerability point of view, it could be maintained that, if there were ironclad outcome data (and there are not, or not yet), all patients should be started on an ARB, and other drugs should only be used if the ARB does not bring the BP into the target range or is not tolerated.**

## Antihypertensive efficacy

Concomitant medications, such as nonsteroidal anti-inflammatory drugs (NSAIDs), or a high salt intake can mitigate the antihypertensive efficacy of certain drug classes, such as ACE inhibitors or ARBs. Beta-blockers have little, if any, effect in isolated systolic hypertension in elderly patients. A high salt intake can counteract the effects of diuretics and blockers of the RAS. In contrast, few, if any, drugs or dietary interventions affect the efficacy of calcium antagonists. Calcium antagonists, of which amlodipine is the prototype, lower BP regardless of age, sex, race, diet, concomitant diseases, or medications. Numerous prospective randomized trials have documented that calcium anatagonists reduce the rate of stroke and heart attack. **From an** efficacy standpoint, the simplistic view could be taken that all patients should be started on a calcium antagonist, as this drug class offers the broadest spectrum of efficacy in all patient populations.

## Cardiovascular protection

From a simplistic, cardioprotective point of view, an ACE inhibitor would clearly be the drug of choice for all patients, as members of this class have shown impressive cardiovascular protection in high-risk patients. Although the BP of black patients responds less well to ACE inhibitor therapy, and the risk of angioedema is several times higher than in white patients, ACE inhibitors still confer a distinct nephroprotective effect.

## Economic considerations

From a purely economical point of view (which may be the most simplistic of all), it could be maintained that therapy for all patients should begin with a low dose of a thiazide diuretic and that another drug class should only be used if diuretics are contraindicated, poorly tolerated, or do not lower BP into the target range. This viewpoint is put forward by the JNC 7 guidelines [2] based on the ALLHAT study [19]. Whatever drug class is selected, it must be affordable for the patient. Sophisticated therapeutic wisdom is utterly useless if the patient is unable, or unwilling, to pay for the prescription.

# Chapter 5

# Hypertension as a gateway to cardiovascular risk modification

Measurement of BP is a simple, straightforward procedure that allows us to identify the risk of cardiovascular disease. However, treatment of raised BP is clearly inefficient to reduce the overall associated cardiovascular disease risk. Antihypertensive therapy should, therefore, serve as a gateway to overall cardiovascular risk management and give rise to normal risk estimation. This can be done by using the Framingham risk score [1] or the systems put forward by the European Society of Cardiology [24] and others. We have learned recently that the use of more elaborate risk assessment by a series of biomarkers does not really add much to additional methods of assessing the cardiovascular disease risk. However, one of the most important criticisms of cardiovascular risk estimation is that it is based on limited time projections, most often on 10-year absolute risk estimation. This approach strongly favors treatment of the elderly population because age is a more powerful determinant of the short-term risk in the elderly than in younger patients. Additional risk factors that should be considered are diabetes, decreased GFR, proteinuria and cardiac abnormalities on electrocardiography (ECG). Figure 5 outlines progression of the natural history of hypertensive cardiovascular disease.

A patient is said to be at high risk when he or she has a 10-year Framingham-derived cardiovascular disease risk of 20% or more. Your typical hypertensive male patient, aged 55 or older, will be at this level of risk.

Of note, formal cardiovascular risk disease estimation is no longer necessary for patients with high BP and manifest cardiovascular disease, diabetes or overt end-organ disease. Clearly, these patients are at sufficient risk of cardiovascular disease so that a multifactorial risk factor intervention will be beneficial.

**Range of hypertensive cardiovascular disease from prehypertension to target-organ damage and end-stage disease**

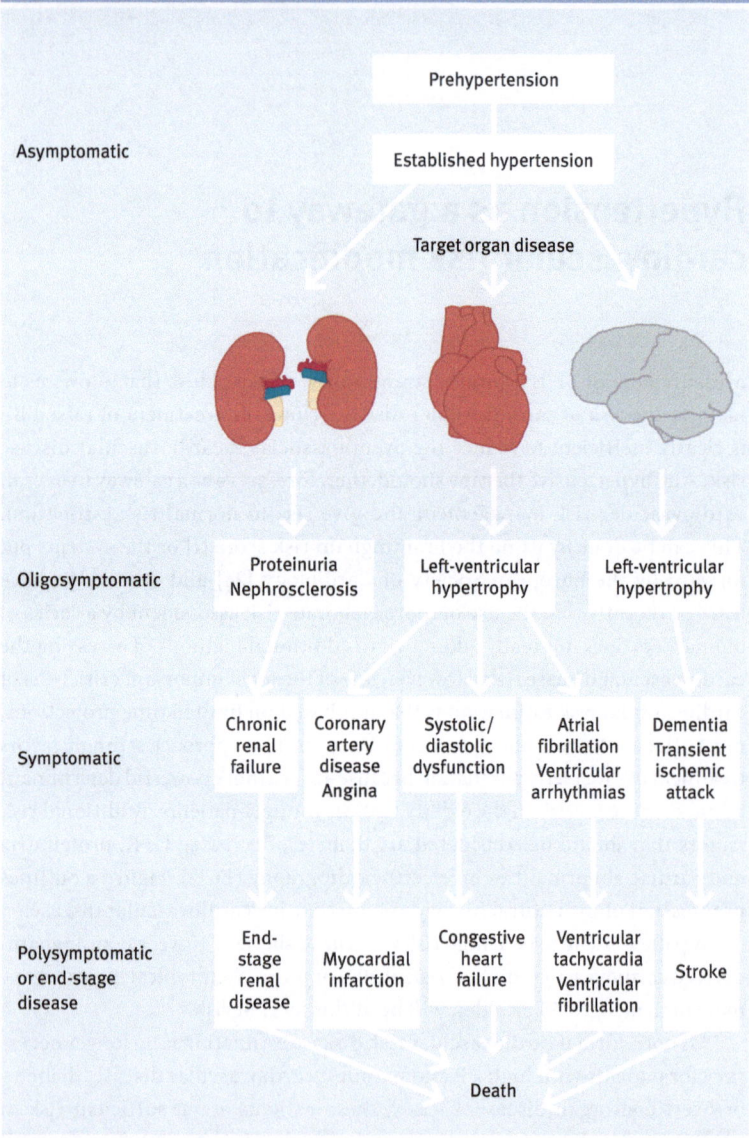

**Figure 5 Range of hypertensive cardiovascular disease from prehypertension to target-organ damage and end-stage disease.** Reproduced with permission from Messerli et al. [25].

# Chapter 6

## To twofer or not to twofer?

The two-for-one therapeutic concept or, namely, to treat two conditions with one drug, is attractive for a variety of reasons; among these are a reduction in adverse effects, the number of pills, and cost. Physicians and patients, therefore, like the "twofer" and use it whenever possible. Unfortunately, the concept of the twofer has never been vigorously tested. Ironclad trials have shown that beta-blockers confer secondary cardioprotection in patients who have suffered an acute MI [26]. However, beta-blockers have no primary cardioprotective effect in hypertension, and there are no studies showing that the reduction of BP by beta-blockers confers any additional benefit in the post-MI patient with hypertension, as would be expected from the fact that two risk factors are modified by one and the same drug. In the post-MI patient, it seems more logical to use a beta-blocker for secondary cardioprotection and to treat hypertension separately by adding another drug class that has been shown to have outcome benefits in hypertension, such as a diuretic, calcium antagonist, or ACE inhibitor. The twofer, however, is perfectly acceptable in the same situation for the ACE inhibitor. ACE inhibitors have well-documented benefits in the post-MI patient (secondary prevention) [27,28], and the treatment of hypertension with an ACE inhibitor has been shown to reduce morbidity and mortality (primary prevention). Therefore, an ACE inhibitor is an excellent twofer for cardioprotection and for treatment of hypertension in the post-MI patient. Similarly, in the patient with hypertension and heart failure, an ACE inhibitor (or an ARB) should be the drug of choice because these agents have well-documented benefits in both heart failure and hypertension. Treatment with a drug that blocks the RAS will lower morbidity and mortality.

A twofer is also very much acceptable if it serves to improve symptoms and signs of a comorbid condition in a patient with hypertension. For instance, a thiazide diuretic has been shown to diminish the risk of osteoporosis in elderly patients. Calcium antagonists, particularly verapamil, may have a beneficial effect on migraine headaches. Nonselective beta-blockers may favorably affect familial tremor. ACE inhibitors or ARBs diminish diuretic-associated potassium loss and insulin resistance. Postsynaptic alpha-blockers diminish nocturia and symptoms of prostatism in patients with benign prostatic hypertrophy, but may increase the risk of heart failure. As heart failure is a very common cardiac endstage of hypertensive cardiovascular disease, alpha-blockers should be avoided as first-line antihypertensive drugs. As attractive as the twofer is, before using it extensively, knowledge of outcome data in hypertensive cardiovascular disease is needed (ie, whether the drug class has been documented to improve the symptoms or morbidity and mortality of the comorbid condition). Figure 6 lists some currently acceptable twofers. It is also worth remembering that some antihypertensive drugs may have unfavorable effects on comorbid conditions, as outlined in Figure 7.

| Favorable effects of certain drugs on comorbid conditions | |
| --- | --- |
| Angina | Beta-blockers, calcium antagonists |
| Myocardial infarction | Beta-blockers, non-DHP calcium antagonists, ACE inhibitors |
| Osteoporosis | Thiazide diuretics |
| Atrial fibrillation | |
| • Rate control | Beta-blockers, non-DHP calcium antagonists |
| • Prevention | ACE inhibitors, ARBs |
| Heart failure | Beta-blockers (carvedilol), ACE inhibitors, ARBs |
| Impaired renal function | ACE inhibitors, ARBs |
| Diabetes mellitus (types 1 and 2) with proteinuria | ACE inhibitors, ARBs, calcium antagonists |
| Dyslipidemia | Alpha-blockers |
| Migraine | Beta-blockers (noncardioselective), non-DHP calcium antagonists |
| Hyperthyroidism | Beta-blockers |
| Essential tremor | Beta-blockers (noncardioselective) |
| Cyclosporine-induced hypertension | DHP-calcium antagonists |
| Prostatism | Alpha-blockers |
| Erectile dysfunction | ARBs |
| Hyperuricemia | Losartan |

Figure 6 Favorable effects of certain drugs on comorbid conditions. ACE, angiotensin-converting enzyme; ARBs, angiotensin receptor blockers; DHP, dihydropyridine.

## Unfavorable effects of certain drugs on comorbid conditions

| | |
|---|---|
| Erectile dysfunction | Beta-blockers, diuretics, antiadrenergics |
| Heart failure | Calcium antagonist (except amlodipine) |
| Renal failure | Potassium-sparing agents, ACE inhibitors, ARBs, thiazide diuretics |
| Renovascular disease | ACE inhibitors, ARBs, thiazide diuretics |
| Peripheral vascular disease | Beta-blockers* |
| Second- or third-degree heart block | Beta-blockers, non-DHP calcium antagonists |
| Diabetes mellitus (types 1 and 2) | Beta-blockers*, high-dose diuretics |
| Dyslipidemia | Beta-blockers*, diuretics (high dose) |
| Gout | Diuretics |
| Bronchospastic disease | Beta-blockers |
| Pregnancy | ACE inhibitors, ARBs |
| Depression | Beta-blockers, antiadrenergics, reserpine |

**Figure 7 Unfavorable effects of certain drugs on comorbid conditions.** *Carvedilol and nebivolol have less metabolic adverse effects than other beta blockers. ACE, angiotensin-converting enzyme; ARBs, angiotensin receptor blockers; DHP, dihydropyridine.

# Chapter 7

# When initial therapy is insufficient – To uptitrate, to substitute, or to combine?

One of the most common questions practicing physicians face after starting a patient on treatment with a given antihypertensive drug is how to proceed when BP remains elevated. That physicians are uneasy with this question is illustrated by the fact that patients are often treated for years with the same dose of the same drug or combination, despite the fact that BP is not at goal. Any excuses volunteered by the patient (ie, crowded parking garage, mother-in-law visiting) seem good enough to rationalize that day's high BP as an exception and delay further therapeutic intervention.

The decision as to which of the three options (to uptitrate, to substitute, or to combine) is best for a given patient can often be based on a few simple facts pertaining to the efficacy and side effects of various drugs.

## Uptitration

Uptitration of the original drug to double the dosage is reasonable only if distinctly enhanced antihypertensive efficacy has been documented and the cost is not prohibitive. Most antihypertensive drugs have a rather shallow dose–response curve and increasing the dose has little additional effect on BP. For instance, doubling the starting dose of losartan from 50 mg to 100 mg, has not been shown to increase antihypertensive efficacy. In a situation like this, it is more rational to combine a low dose of a diuretic with the ARB. Indeed, the combination has been shown to lower BP better than a higher dose of losartan monotherapy [29].

In contrast, additional antihypertensive efficacy can be gained using amlodipine when the starting dose is doubled from 5 mg to 10 mg; furthermore, the cost of the 10 mg dose is less than that of two 5 mg doses. However, the incidence of pedal edema also increases with the higher dose of amlodipine. Pedal edema is a well-known, dose-dependent side effect of all dihydropyridine calcium antagonists (Figure 8) [23,30]. In a middle-aged, overweight woman, it is probably not a good idea to uptitrate to 10 mg of amlodipine because the likelihood of her experiencing pedal edema is substantial.

As can be seen in Figure 8, uptitration from 15 mg to 20 mg does not increase antihypertensive efficacy but doubles the occurrence of pedal edema.

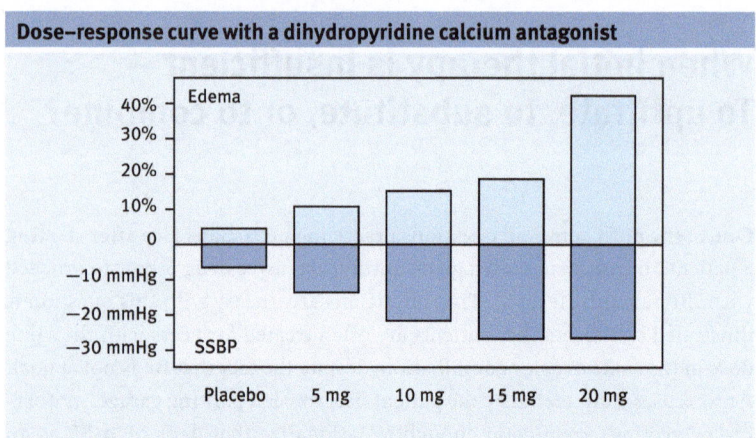

**Figure 8 Dose–response curve with a dihydropyridine calcium antagonist.** CR, controlled release; SSBP, supine systolic blood pressure. Adapted from Chrysant et al. [30].

## Combination

In contrast, the combination of an ACE inhibitor or an ARB with a calcium antagonist has been shown to diminish the incidence of pedal edema [23]. Unlike the pedal edema seen with calcium antagonists, the cough seen with ACE inhibitors is not dose dependent. If a patient does not exhibit a cough with 1 mg of trandolapril, it is unlikely that there will be a cough with 8 mg of trandolapril. Therefore, uptitration can be pursued without much concern. The only common dose-dependent side effects from ACE inhibitors (and to a lesser extent ARBs) is hyperkalemia and a decrease in GFR in susceptible patients.

The above considerations make it clear that, as a general rule, it may be better to combine than to uptitrate monotherapy to the maximum dose. Uptitration to maximal dose, or higher, should be considered if dose-dependent adverse effects are absent, or tolerable, and if the dose pricing curve is flat. A recent meta-analysis of 11,000 participants from 42 trials reported that the incremental BP reduction achieved from combining drugs from two different classes was approximately five times greater than doubling the dose of one drug. Combination should therefore be preferred over uptitration [31].

## Substitution

Substituting a different antihypertensive drug should be considered if there is no antihypertensive efficacy with a reasonable dose, as is occasionally seen with beta-blockers, ACE inhibitors or ARBs in black patients, or if there are intolerable side effects, such as angioedema. Fortunately, most modern antihypertensive drugs are well tolerated and serious adverse effects are few. Some patients are even willing to put up with a scratchy throat or low-grade cough associated with ACE inhibitors, or the pedal edema associated with calcium antagonists, once they know that these are harmless conditions related to the drugs.

# Chapter 8

# How aggressively should blood pressure be lowered?

The VALUE study clearly established that patients whose BP was under control after 6 months had a much lower risk of heart attack and stroke than did patients whose BP remained elevated [32]. This appears to indicate that swift BP control should be achieved and argues against the old dictum of "start low, go slow." It should be considered, however, that in the VALUE study most patients were taken off multiple drugs and were put on monotherapy (ie, valsartan 80 mg) for several months. Clearly, this is not the way a practicing physician would treat patients. In most placebo-controlled antihypertensive trials, the Kaplan–Meier curves of morbidity and mortality grow apart after 6 months to 1 year. It seems reasonable to treat elevated BP aggressively in a younger patient whose cardiovascular system can tolerate an abrupt decrease in BP. In such a patient, antihypertensive therapy may be initiated with two drugs, such as an ARB and a diuretic, or a calcium antagonist and an ACE inhibitor. However, in an elderly, more fragile patient, it is probably justified to start on monotherapy and to uptitrate gradually every 4–6 weeks.

## Blood pressure lowering in normotensive patients

The Framingham study has clearly documented that, even within the normotensive range, patients with higher BPs have a higher risk of cardiovascular morbidity than those who have an optimal BP [1]. This raises the question of whether one should consider antihypertensive therapy in normotensive patients. Indeed, several studies have shown that lowering BP in the so-called normotensive population reduces cardiovascular morbidity and mortality. This is particularly true for stroke but less so for coronary heart disease. Although it has been accepted that lipid lowering in high-risk patients is beneficial regardless of lipid levels, the same principle is still somewhat foreign with regard to antihypertensive therapy.

In my opinion, some normotensive patients at high cardiovascular risk may benefit from antihypertensive therapy. In fact, the benefits of antihypertensive therapy in these normotensive patients will probably exceed those seen in mildly hypertensive patients without any significant risk factors. However, special attention should be paid to patients with coronary artery disease and low diastolic BP levels (see Chapter 2).

## Blood pressure lowering in prehypertensive patients

The JNC created a new BP class in 2003 called prehypertension [2]. The issue surrounding this entity has stirred tempers to an extent that seems more suitable to medieval theologians than to modern scientists. The extensively quoted meta-analysis of Lewington [33] suggested a continuous relationship between the risk of cardiovascular disease (stroke, coronary heart disease, and vascular disease) and usual BP values down to at least 115/75 mmHg. In the Framingham cohort [1], an increase in cardiovascular events was reported in individuals with a higher baseline BP within the normotensive range (ie, below 140/90 mmHg). In this cohort of normotensive subjects, BP levels paralleled cardiovascular disease risk in the same way as they did in hypertension. It follows that normotensive individuals with a host of additional risk factors could be at higher overall cardiovascular risk than patients without risk factors with mild hypertension. It follows further that the absolute benefits of antihypertensive treatment for such normotensive subjects could be greater than for patients with uncomplicated hypertension. Irrespective of BP levels, it is always preferable to bring BP to goal by nonpharmacologic means if possible. The experienced clinician has learned that patients' adherence to lifestyle intervention is notoriously poor. Thus, even in some normotensive individuals, antihypertensive therapy may have to be considered. When weighing the pros and cons, we should consider that the benefits in this population are fairly small, and therefore the long-term safety of any drug used has to be well documented. The only drug classes that fulfill these criteria are the ARBs [34] and possibly some calcium antagonists. Diuretics and beta-blockers elicit metabolic side effects that make them unsuitable for the treatment of patients with prehypertension [35].

# Chapter 9

# Evidence-based versus eminence-based therapy

Eminence-based therapy can be defined as *"making the same mistakes with increasing confidence over an impressive number of years"* [36]. Numerous prospective, randomized large trials have taught us what is now defined as evidence-based medicine (EBM) in the treatment of hypertension. However, a critical analysis of these trials remains extremely important because they provide the results that should be translated into clinical practice. For instance, the SHEP program [18] is commonly used as EBM for the safety and efficacy of diuretics in patients with isolated systolic hypertension. Before applying this evidence to an individual patient, however, the physician should remember that out of 100 screened patients with isolated systolic hypertension only one was included in the SHEP study and 99 were excluded for one reason or another. Can the evidence derived from 1% of the population be extrapolated to the remaining 99%?

The application of published inclusion criteria from 13 randomized clinical trials in the elderly to a patient cohort of 5530 patients with hypertension who were over the age of 60 years and recruited from general practices, showed that a total of 71.3% of these patients met at least one exclusion criterion [37]. This clearly indicates that trial-eligible patients are remarkably healthy compared with those who are excluded (Figure 9).

In my opinion, EBM never seems to quite apply to the patient sitting in front of me and, as clinicians, we will have to continue to make seemingly arbitrary decisions in everyday practice.

| Eligibility for participation in clinical trials among 5530 elderly patients, according to criteria from 13 trials involving elderly patients with hypertension | | | |
|---|---|---|---|
| Variable | Ineligible patients | Eligible patients | *p*-Value |
| No. of patients (%) | 3944 (71.3) | 1586 (28.7) | – |
| Mean age (years)* | 69.3±6.4 | 67.1±5.8 | <0.001 |
| Female sex (%) | 57.0 | 62.8 | <0.001 |
| Family history of early CV disease (%) | 34.7 | 22.1 | <0.001 |
| Dyslipidemia (%) | 76.3 | 71.4 | <0.001 |
| Abdominal obesity (%) | 61.7 | 55.4 | <0.001 |
| Left ventricular hypertrophy (%) | 37.5 | 21.5 | <0.001 |
| Coronary heart disease (%) | 49.2 | 19.1 | <0.001 |
| Heart failure (%) | 20.0 | 2.1 | <0.01 |

Figure 9 Eligibility for participation in clinical trials among 5530 elderly patients, according to criteria from 13 trials involving elderly patients with hypertension. *means ±SD. CV, cardiovascular. Reproduced with permission from Messerli et al. [37].

# Chapter 10

## Combination therapy

Cardiovascular risk factors, such as hypertension, diabetes, and hyperlipidemia, as well as cardiovascular disease states, such as coronary heart disease, heart failure, and certain arrhythmias, are amenable to a variety of therapeutic interventions that have been proven to be beneficial. However, the combination of these interventions has rarely been studied in a rigorous scientific way. No data are available that analyze the relevant contribution of each drug to the overall outcome in a given patient. Progress has been made in identifying and understanding some drug interactions, allowing the rational combination of certain drugs in a given patient. Drug combinations may be rational for several reasons (Figure 10):

- Drug A may enhance the efficacy of Drug B. Such an additive effect is the most common reason for combining two drugs in one patient. If BP or low-density lipoprotein (LDL) cholesterol do not fall to target levels with monotherapy, it is reasonable to consider adding another drug that, hopefully, will get the levels closer to target.

- Drug A is effective but has an adverse effect or elicits a risk that can be antagonized or abolished by Drug B; Drug B may or may not have an effect on a surrogate end point. A classic example of this scenario is the use of a potassium-sparing diuretic, such as triamterene, with HCTZ. The efficacy of triamterene with regard to BP is negligible, but it diminishes the potassium depletion caused by the thiazide diuretic. In contrast, the addition of spironolactone, or eplerenone, to HCTZ confers distinct additional antihypertensive efficacy and also a potassium-retaining effect.

- Drug A is effective for one risk factor and Drug B is effective for another risk factor of the same disease state; both of these risk factors are common in a high percentage of the population. An example of this scenario is the combination of an antihypertensive drug (amlodipine) with an ACE inhibitor or a statin. In addition, both of these drugs may have an effect on endothelial function that, potentially, could be additive or synergistic. By putting two drugs into one pill, adherence to therapy can be improved and, hopefully, morbidity and mortality will be reduced in an additive way. Fixed combinations of aspirin with beta-blockers, ACE inhibitors, or statins certainly would improve compliance in post-MI patients. However, if improvement of compliance is the only reason for use, the drawbacks and disadvantages of combination therapy may well outweigh its benefits. What then are the potential pitfalls of combination therapy?

- By initiating two drugs at the same time, nonspecific adverse events cannot be pinpointed to a specific agent. In general, class-specific side effects, such as cough with ACE inhibitors and pedal edema with dihydropyridine calcium antagonists, can be clearly attributed to the specific drug. However, this is much more difficult with adverse effects such as dizziness, nausea, headaches, and flushing.

- The busy practicing physician may, occasionally, not remember the ingredients of the fixed combination and add a fixed combination to monotherapy in a patient who is already on one of the two components.

The above considerations make it clear that the most important rationale for combining two drugs into one pill is to increase efficacy and, to a lesser extent, diminish adverse effects.

| Suggested matrix of combination therapy | | | | | | |
|---|---|---|---|---|---|---|
| | Diuretics | Beta-blockers | Non-DHP CCB | DHP CCB | ACE inhibitors | ARBs |
| Beta-blockers | G | | | | | |
| Non-DHP CCB | G | P | | | | |
| DHP CCB | F | G | F | | | |
| ACE inhibitors | G | F | G | G | | |
| ARBs | G | F | G | G | P | |
| DRI | G | F | G | G | F | F |

Figure 10 **Suggested matrix of combination therapy.** ACE, angiotensin-converting enzyme; ARB, angiotensin receptor blocker; CCB, calcium channel blocker; DHP, dihydropyridine; DRI, direct renin inhibitor; F, fair; G, good; P, poor.

## Drug interactions

Drug–drug interactions have become increasingly important over the past few decades because, in most cases, two or more drugs are needed to get BP to goal, and also because hypertension is rarely an isolated disorder and concomitant risk factors or diseases may require multiple drugs that can, potentially, interact with a given antihypertensive agent. It is almost impossible for the practicing physician to remember all potential interactions, some of which can lead to severe and even fatal adverse events. Fortunately, computer programs, such as Epocrates®, have become very useful in identifying the most important interactions. Of particular interest is the long list of drugs or agents that interfere with the cytochrome P450 system. An example of such an agent is grapefruit juice, which has been shown to increase plasma concentration of certain calcium antagonists and statins. All other factors being equal (which they rarely are), the practicing physician is advised to preferentially use a drug with less potential for interaction; that is, one not metabolized by the cytochrome system. From this point of view, amlodipine is a better choice than verapamil, and eprosartan a better choice than losartan.

## Diuretics and diuretic combinations

Fixed combinations of a thiazide diuretic and a potassium-sparing drug are commonly used as initial therapy for the treatment of hypertension. In the USA, there are three such fixed combinations available (Figure 11). Of note, triamterene and amiloride have relatively little diuretic or antihypertensive effect, whereas spironolactone and eplerenone act synergistically on BP.

| Fixed-dose diuretic combinations |
|---|
| Amiloride 5 or 2.5 mg/HCTZ 50 mg |
| Spironolactone 25 or 50 mg/HCTZ 50 or 25 mg |
| Triamterene 37.5, 50, or 75 mg/HCTZ 25 or 50 mg |
| Triameterene 50 mg/benzthiazide 25 mg |

Figure 11 **Fixed-dose diuretic combinations.** HCTZ, hydrochlorothiazide.

These compounds serve mainly to retain the potassium that is excessively excreted with thiazide diuretics. In contrast, spironolactone, an aldosterone antagonist, has been shown to lower BP and also to exert some diuretic effects. The prevention of hypokalemia with thiazide diuretics is important because, as shown in the SHEP study [12], hypokalemia may remove the benefits conferred by the decrease in BP. In addition, the risk of sudden death has been shown to rise with increasing doses of thiazide diuretics and to be reduced with the addition of a potassium-sparing compound. In general, fixed diuretic combinations are well tolerated and have remarkably few adverse effects. In combinations containing high doses of ACE inhibitors or ARBs hyperkalemia is of concern in susceptible patients, such as patients with diabetes or chronic renal failure. In rare instances, triamterene has been associated with kidney stones. Spironolactone is known to cause gynecomastia, impotence, menstrual irregularities, and, rarely, agranulocytosis. However, these endocrine adverse effects usually occur at higher doses (above 25 mg/day) only. In the Randomized Aldactone Evaluation Study (RALES) [38], spironolactone was shown to decrease morbidity and mortality when added to standard triple therapy in patients with heart failure. A novel aldosterone antagonist (eplerenone) is available that, while sharing the antihypertensive efficacy of spironolactone, seems to cause less hyperkalemia and few, if any, endocrine abnormalities, such as gynecomastia and menstrual irregularities. Eplerenone seems to be particularly effective in reducing target organ damage, such as left ventricular hypertrophy (LVH) and microproteinuria.

Loop diuretics, such as furosemide and torsemide, can also be combined with potassium-sparing compounds, although no fixed combinations are available. Adverse effects and precautions are similar to those used in combination with the thiazide diuretics.

Occasionally, in therapy-resistant edematous states, the combination of a loop diuretic with a thiazide, such as metolazone, is useful. However, volume depletion and hypokalemia are common adverse effects of this combination and patients need to be monitored closely.

## Beta-blocker and diuretic combinations

Several beta-blocker and diuretic combinations were marketed a number of decades ago when beta-blockers became available in the USA (Figure 12). In most of these fixed combinations, the beta-blocker is combined with 25 mg, or even 50 mg, of HCTZ (or the corresponding dose of a thiazide derivative), a dose that, by today's standard, would have to be considered high. It has been learned that HCTZ doses of 12.5 mg, and even 6.25 mg, lower BP and cause fewer endocrine metabolic adverse effects than the higher doses that were used previously. The dose–response curve with regard to BP plateaus at around 50 mg. However, the dose–response curve with regard to hypokalemia, hyponatremia, hyperuricemia, glucose intolerance, and so on, seems to plateau only at levels of 100–200 mg. Thus, it is in the best interest of the patient to use low-dose diuretics. Indeed, the FDA has approved a very low-dose fixed beta-blocker and diuretic combination (bisoprolol and HCTZ). In this combination, three different dose levels of bisoprolol (2.5 mg, 5 mg, and 10 mg) are combined with only 6.25 mg of HCTZ. The FDA approved this fixed combination for first-line therapy because of solid documentation that it lowered BP more than monotherapy of the same dose of either bisoprolol or HCTZ, and yet all known adverse effects of these two drugs are dose dependent.

## Fixed-dose beta-blocker and diuretic combinations

Atenolol 50 or 100 mg/chlorthalidone 25 mg

Bisoprolol 2.5, 5 or 10 mg/HCTZ 6.25 mg

Metoprolol 50 or 100 mg/HCTZ 25 or 50 mg

Nadolol 40 or 80 mg/bendroflumethiazide 5 mg

Propranolol (extended release) 80, 120 or 160 mg/HCTZ 50 mg

Metoprolol 100 mg/HCTZ 12.5 mg

Propanolol 160 mg/bendrofluazide 5 mg

Timolol 10 mg/bendrofluazide 2.5 mg

Acebutolol 200 mg/HCTZ 12.5 mg

Atenolol 25 mg/bendrofluazide 1.25 mg

Atenolol 50 mg/chlorthalidone 1.25 mg

Oxprenolol 160 mg/cyclopenthiazide 0.25 mg

Pindolol 10 mg/clopamide 5 mg

Figure 12 Fixed-dose beta-blocker and diuretic combinations.

Both beta-blockers and diuretics have been documented to lower BP. The Fifth Report of the JNC, released in 1992, labeled diuretics and beta-blockers as the preferred agents for initial therapy of hypertension. This stand was somewhat softened in 1997 by the JNC VI [39]. Nevertheless, the JNC VI still recommended diuretics and beta-blockers as first-line therapy for uncomplicated hypertension because these were, supposedly, the only two drug classes for which a reduction in morbidity or mortality was shown in hypertension. While this is true for diuretics, it is incorrect for beta-blockers. There is no study in which beta-blockers have been shown to reduce morbidity and mortality in hypertension when compared with placebo. In the large UK Medical Research Council (MRC) study, in patients younger than 65 years of age, diuretics reduced the risk of stroke between two and four times better than beta-blockers, despite an equal fall in BP [40]. One can also estimate from this study that, in order to prevent one heart attack or one stroke by beta-blockade, six patients were made impotent and another seven experienced fatigue to the extent that they decided to withdraw from this therapy. This is hardly a risk/benefit ratio that can be considered acceptable for patients with asymptomatic mild essential hypertension. In JNC 7, thiazide diuretics became the preferred drug class for initial therapy [2].

Does the addition of a beta-blocker to a diuretic enhance the morbidity and mortality benefit of a diuretic? Clearly, the addition of a beta-blocker to a diuretic will lower BP further. However, in the MRC study in elderly patients, whenever a beta-blocker was added to a diuretic, the benefits were diminished, and they vanished completely with beta-blocker monotherapy [40]. Thus, almost in a dose-dependent fashion, the diuretic-induced benefit melted away with an increasing dose of beta-blocker; the more beta-blocker present, the less cardioprotection achieved. Even in the SHEP study, in which many patients received atenolol in addition to baseline diuretic therapy (chlorthalidone), no benefits of this addition were documented [18]. Kostis et al. [41] scrutinized the effects of beta-blocker addition in this study and clearly stated, "*Additional (independent) benefits attributable to atenolol or to reserpine were not identified.*" It seems that most, if not all, benefits, with regard to cardiovascular morbidity and mortality, observed with diuretic and beta-blocker combinations are due to diuretic therapy. As beta-blockers do not have a benign adverse-effect profile, it seems reasonable to avoid a diuretic/ beta-blocker combination for uncomplicated hypertension. This is particularly true for elderly patients, who often present with systolic hypertension. Beta-blockers will reduce heart rate in these patients, which, in turn, leads to a higher stroke volume (ie, an increased amount of blood is ejected into the aorta per heartbeat). This will invariably cause an increase (or a lesser fall) in systolic pressure and a decrease in diastolic pressure. The simple rule to remember is that bradycardia causes systolic hypertension.

It must be emphasized that there are well-documented indications for beta-blockers; these include certain disease states, such as the post-MI patient with hypertension or the patient with heart failure. In the Carvedilol or Metoprolol European Trial (COMET) – the largest trial to date to be carried out in patients with heart failure – carvedilol was shown to reduce cardio-vascular morbidity and mortality better than metoprolol [42]. Numerous studies, carried out 25 years ago, have shown that beta-blockers reduce morbidity and mortality, mostly by reducing reinfarction and sudden death in the post-MI patient. However, in a contemporary patient population, this was only demonstrated with carvedilol. Should such a patient have hypertension, or become hypertensive in the post-MI time period, the addition of a low-dose thiazide diuretic to the beta-blocker must be considered a logical therapeutic step. Similarly, in heart failure, beta-blockers and diuretics are a cornerstone of the therapeutic strategy and should be combined in a fixed combination whenever possible. Commonly, physicians fear that they will lose some therapeutic flexibility when using fixed combinations. This is certainly true with regard to downtitration, but not necessarily for uptitration. Thus, there is nothing wrong in telling a patient who is on a fixed diuretic and beta-blocker combination to occasionally take an additional dose of a diuretic if he or she is exposed to an inappropriate dietary salt load. In unstable clinical situations, as a rule, fixed combinations should be avoided.

## Antiadrenergic and diuretic combinations

Diuretic and antiadrenergic combinations were common a few years ago, but are sparingly used in this day and age. Most contain fairly high doses of diuretics and some have to be given twice a day (Figure 13). Antiadrenergic drugs, such as methyldopa, clonidine, guanabenz, and even reserpine, have a favorable effect on a variety of pathophysiologic findings of hypertensive cardiovascular disease. These drugs reduce LVH, vascular hypertrophy, vascular resistance, and proteinuria, maintain cardiac output, and preserve renal hemodynamics. Even in patients with metabolic syndrome, antiadrenergic drugs exert a favorable effect on abnormal endocrine metabolic findings. In low doses, these drugs are reasonably well tolerated. Unfortunately, at the dose at which their antihypertensive efficacy equals that of other drug classes, their adverse-effect profile often prohibits their use in patients with mild hypertension. The most common adverse effects are fatigue, depression, sexual dysfunction (in men and women), cognitive dysfunction, weird dreams, and nightmares. Combination with a low-dose diuretic enhances the antihypertensive efficacy and has no effect on the side-effect profile.

It is, therefore, often possible to "get away" with the combination of a low-dose diuretic and a low-dose antiadrenergic drug. No morbidity and mortality studies in hypertension have shown that either monotherapy of an antiadrenergic drug or the addition of an antiadrenergic drug to diuretic therapy will reduce morbidity and mortality.

| Fixed-dose antiadrenergic drug and diuretic combinations |
| --- |
| Clonidine 0.1, 0.2, or 0.3 mg/chlorthalidone 15 mg |
| Methyldopa 250 or 500 mg/HCTZ 15, 25, 30, or 50 mg |

Figure 13 **Fixed-dose antiadrenergic drug and diuretic combinations.** HCTZ, hydrochlorothiazide.

## Calcium antagonist and diuretic combinations

The general clinical contention that a diuretic should not be combined with a calcium antagonist, unless there is edema caused by calcium antagonist monotherapy, is wrong for several reasons. In the early 1980s, an uncontrolled study in a small number of patients showed that the addition of a diuretic to verapamil had no additive effect on BP. Ever since this study, physicians have been reluctant to combine a diuretic with a calcium antagonist, dihydropyridine or not. However, several large, double-blind, factorial design studies have clearly documented that, as with other combinations, there is an additive effect on BP with the combination of diuretics and calcium antagonists, more so with the nondihydropyridines than the dihydropyridines. Thus, from a BP point of view, there is little reason not to add a calcium antagonist to a diuretic, or vice versa. Of some concern may be the fact that diuretics cause hypokalemia, and calcium antagonists, although not known to directly cause hypokalemia, also have some natriuretic effects. Thus, the combination of the two could theoretically result in excessive fluid volume depletion. As there are no well-controlled studies in this area, it is unknown whether this concern is indeed real.

Calcium antagonists, particularly the dihydropyridines, commonly cause pedal edema. Most physicians' knee jerk response when presented with pedal edema is to add a diuretic. However, the pedal edema seen with the use of calcium antagonists is not caused by salt and water retention, but by intra-capillary hypertension secondary to the diminished arteriolar vasoconstriction with upright posture. Thus, this form of vasodilatory edema responds poorly to diuretic therapy, but very well to blockade of the RAS, either by an ACE inhibitor or an ARB. The fact that no fixed combination of a calcium antagonist and a diuretic is available indicates that pharmaceutical companies seem to be reluctant, for good reason or not, to tackle this issue.

## Calcium antagonist and beta-blocker combinations

In the USA, no fixed combination of a calcium antagonist with a beta-blocker is available. However, in Europe, at least one such combination is on the market and has been quite successful. Short-acting calcium antagonists are well known to produce cardio-acceleration, an increase in heart rate and cardiac output, and sympathetic stimulation. With the long-acting, once-a-day agents, cardio-acceleration and sympathetic stimulation are minimal but can still be documented with some dihydropyridine calcium antagonists, even after weeks of monotherapy. In contrast, long-term therapy with the long-acting nondihydro-pyridine agents verapamil and diltiazem leads to a fall in sympathetic activity. The increase in sympathetic activity, however small, with dihydropyridine calcium antagonists can be counteracted by the addition of a beta-blocker. Therefore, the combination of these two drug classes seems useful, not only in hypertension but also in patients with stable coronary disease. Both beta-blockers and dihydropyridine calcium antagonists have benefits in patients with coronary disease; the negative effects of the calcium antagonist can be diminished by concomitant beta-blockade. In one morbidity and mortality study, such a combination was shown to be beneficial in patients with coronary heart disease. In contrast to dihydropyridine calcium antagonists, verapamil and diltiazem should not be combined with beta-blockers; this is because of additive effects on sinus node and atrioventricular conduction.

## Beta-blockers with either ACE inhibitors or ARBs

No fixed combination is available of a beta-blocker with either an ACE inhibitor or an ARB, indicating that there is little interest in developing such a combination. Indeed, there are some reasons to suspect that such a combination may have a distinctly less-than-additive effect on BP; this viewpoint is supported by the ALLHAT study [43]. Although beta-blockers have been available for the treatment of hypertension for a number of decades, the mechanism of their antihypertensive effect is still ill understood. To some extent, it seems to be related to a decrease in renin secretion from juxtaglomerular cells. A decrease in renin secretion means that there is less angiotensin I available for conversion to angiotensin II. As a consequence, an ACE inhibitor will have less substrate to work on, which, obviously, would translate into a diminished efficacy. The same reasoning holds true for the ARB, as beta-blockade will diminish the levels of circulating angiotensin II, and so the ARB will exert less efficacy in blocking the angiotensin II receptor.

However, with ACE inhibition or angiotensin receptor blockade, juxtaglomerular cells become stimulated and more renin is secreted because of the lack of biofeedback. This "compensatory" renin secretion could be blunted by the addition of a beta-blocker. Conceivably, therefore, the beta-blocker could have additional antihypertensive efficacy by diminishing circulating renin levels in patients who are either on an ACE inhibitor or an ARB. In some studies, an additional antihypertensive effect has been demonstrated when a beta-blocker was added to an ACE inhibitor. However, the efficacy of such combination therapy was not tested in the upper dose range of either drug class. It is, therefore, difficult to judge whether or not there are additive effects of the two drug classes.

The issue is completely different for heart failure. Ever since the Cooperative North Scandinavian Enalapril Survival Study (CONSENSUS) [44], ACE inhibitors have been a cornerstone in the management of patients with heart failure. Numerous studies have documented that beta-blockade or, alpha/beta-blockade, as documented with carvedilol in COMET [45], also exerts a beneficial effect in these patients, whether they are taking an ACE inhibitor or not. Beta-blockers exert their beneficial effects, at least to some extent, by shielding the heart and the whole cardiovascular system from surges in catecholamines. Circulating catecholamines are known to be one of the most powerful prognosticators in patients with heart failure. Conversely, ACE inhibitors are probably beneficial, not only by unloading the heart, but also by diminishing the detrimental effects of circulating angiotensin. Thus, in heart failure, the effects of beta-blockers and ACE inhibitors, or ARBs, are distinctly different from each other. The Valsartan Heart Failure Trial (Val-HeFT) [46] has shown that ARBs (valsartan) can also be combined with beta-blockers and that this combination will result in an improved outcome. Whether or not a triple combination (eg, a beta-blocker, an ACE inhibitor, and an ARB), may be advisable is currently hotly debated. Although, as the morbidity of such patients was reduced in the Candesartan in Heart Failure Assessment of Reduction in Mortality and Morbidity (CHARM) study when compared with dual combinations of either drug class, there were no observed effects on mortality [46]. The safety issue of triple combination therefore remains unresolved.

Similar to heart failure patients, the post-MI patient will greatly benefit from the combination of a beta-blocker and an ACE inhibitor. This combination has been shown to reduce remodeling and to prevent recurrent MI, sudden death, and heart failure in these patients. Ongoing studies should establish the role of ARBs in combination with beta-blockers for this indication.

In summary, it seems reasonable to combine a beta-blocker with an ACE inhibitor (or an ARB) in patients with left ventricular dysfunction or heart failure, or those having suffered an MI. However, such a combination may be less useful in patients with uncomplicated hypertension.

## ACE inhibitor and diuretic combinations

Numerous fixed combinations of ACE inhibitors and diuretics are presently on the market (Figure 14). Almost all ACE inhibitors available can also be found in fixed combinations with HCTZ. There are several reasons for the popularity of ACE inhibitor and diuretic combinations:

- In many factorial design studies, the combination has been shown to clearly be additive with regard to BP. Thus, the combination provides further antihypertensive efficacy than either of the two drugs in monotherapy.

- The addition of a diuretic to the ACE inhibitor prolongs the antihypertensive efficacy. Captopril, when given as monotherapy, should be dosed at least twice, but better three times, a day in order to achieve a smooth antihypertensive efficacy throughout a 24-hour period. However, when captopril is combined with HCTZ and given once daily, it has been shown to lower BP over a full 24-hour period. The FDA has recognized this efficacy-prolonging effect of combination therapy by allowing the fixed combination of captopril and HCTZ to be marketed as a once-a-day, fixed combination. The FDA has allowed this fixed combination to be used as initial therapy for the treatment of uncomplicated hypertension.

- Diuretics produce fluid volume depletion and thereby stimulate the RAS and, to a lesser extent, the sympathetic nervous system. Stimulation of the RAS is prone to counteract the diuretic-induced fall in BP. Thus, a blockade of this system by an ACE inhibitor will antagonize this compensatory effect and lead to a further increase in antihypertensive efficacy.

- Diuretics are known to cause potassium depletion and to cause some degree of insulin resistance and glucose intolerance. ACE inhibitors are known to antagonize these effects. Particularly important is the antagonism of the two drugs with regard to potassium. In the SHEP study, patients with hypokalemia had no reduction in cardiovascular morbid events, despite a similar fall in BP to that seen in normokalemic patients [12]. Thus, hypokalemia in patients taking diuretics will abolish the beneficial effects of a fall in BP. The addition of an ACE inhibitor in these patients is prone to diminish the kaluretic effects, to restore potassium homeostasis and, thereby, to enhance the benefits of diuretic therapy. Hyperuricemia, a common adverse effect of diuretic therapy, is also influenced favorably by the addition of an ACE inhibitor. ACE inhibitors increase renal blood flow to some extent and, as renal blood flow is a determinant of uric acid excretion, an ACE inhibitor will, in general, have a small hypouricemic effect. Some studies have identified uric acid as an independent cardiovascular

| Fixed-dose ACE inhibitor and diuretic combinations |
|---|
| Benazepril 5, 10, or 20 mg/HCTZ 6.25, 12.5, or 25 mg |
| Captopril 25 or 50 mg/HCTZ 15 or 25 mg |
| Enalapril 5, 10, or 20 mg/HCTZ 12.5 or 25 mg |
| Lisinopril 10 or 20 mg/HCTZ 12.5 mg or 25 mg |
| Perindopril 2 mg/indapamide 6.25 mg |

**Figure 14 Fixed-dose ACE inhibitor and diuretic combinations.** ACE, angiotensin-converting enzyme inhibitor; HCTZ, hydrochlorothiazide.

risk factor; however, there is no study showing that a reduction of uric acid by pharmacologic therapy would improve outcome.

The dose of HCTZ most often used in fixed combination with ACE inhibitors is 12.5 mg. Occasionally, 25 mg combinations are also available. Although both drug classes (diuretics and ACE inhibitors) have been shown to reduce morbidity and mortality in hypertension, there is no study showing that the combination has an additive effect in this regard. Importantly, the ACCOMPLISH study teaches us that an ACE inhibitor/HCTZ combination reduces morbidity and mortality significantly less well than a combination of the same ACE inhibitor with amlodipine.

## ARB and diuretic combinations

Numerous fixed combinations of ARBs and diuretics are presently on the market (Figure 15). Almost all available ARBs can be found in fixed combination with HCTZ. As with ACE inhibitor and diuretic combinations, there are several reasons for the popularity of ARB and diuretic combinations:

- In some studies, the combination has been shown to be additive with regard to BP. Thus, the combination provides further antihypertensive efficacy than either of the two drugs in monotherapy.
- Diuretics produce fluid volume depletion and, thereby, stimulate the RAS and, to a lesser extent, the sympathetic nervous system. Stimulation of the RAS is prone to counteract the diuretic-induced fall in BP. Thus, a blockade of this system by an ARB will antagonize this compensatory effect and lead to a further increase in antihypertensive efficacy.
- Diuretics are known to cause potassium depletion and some degree of insulin resistance and glucose intolerance. ARBs are known to antagonize these effects. Particularly important is the antagonism of the two drugs with regard to potassium. In the SHEP study [12], patients who had hypokalemia had no reduction in cardiovascular morbid events, despite a similar fall in BP as patients who were normokalemic. Thus, hypokalemia in patients taking diuretics will abolish the beneficial effects of a fall in BP. The addition of an ARB in these patients is prone to diminish the kaluretic effects, to restore potassium homeostasis and, thereby, to enhance the benefits of diuretic therapy.
- Diuretics are known to increase uric acid levels and, occasionally, to precipitate a gout attack in susceptible patients. Drugs that increase renal blood flow are known to have a slight uricosuric effect. Thus, in general, the addition of an ARB to a diuretic will lower uric acid to some extent. However, in contrast to all other ARBs, losartan has been shown to have a distinct hypouricemic effect. The combination of losartan with a diuretic almost diminishes the

hyperuricemic effect of the diuretic. This antagonism occurs with both fixed combinations of losartan and HCTZ (50 mg/12.5 mg and 100 mg/25 mg). Thus, in a patient whose baseline uric acid is at the upper limit of normal, losartan may be the preferred ARB to add to HCTZ. Nevertheless, patients should be warned that such fixed combination treatment could still precipitate a gout attack with certain dietary excesses. Lowering of uric acid may not only be important as a preventive measure for gout, but also carry independent benefits for cardiovascular risk factors. Hyperuricemia has been identified in many, but not all, studies as an independent risk factor for cardiovascular morbidity and mortality. No study has shown that the lowering of uric acid improves the cardiovascular risk. However, all other things being equal (which they rarely ever are), it stands to reason that most physicians prefer to see a lower, rather than a higher, uric acid level in their patients.

### Fixed-dose ARB and diuretic combinations

Candesartan 16 mg/HCTZ 12.5 mg

Eprosartan 600 mg/HCTZ 12.5 or 25 mg

Irbesartan 150 or 300 mg/HCTZ 12.5 mg

Losartan 50 or 100 mg/HCTZ 12.5 or 25 mg

Valsartan 80 or 160 mg/HCTZ 12.5 or 25 mg

Olmesartan 20 or 40 mg/HCTZ 12.5 or 25 mg

Telmisartan 40 or 80 mg/HCTZ 12.5 or 25 mg

**Figure 15 Fixed-dose ARB and diuretic combinations.** ARB, angiotensin receptor blocker; HCTZ, hydrochlorothiazide.

The dose of HCTZ most often used in fixed combination with ARBs is 12.5 mg; 25 mg combinations are also available. Although both drug classes (diuretics and ARBs) have been shown to reduce morbidity and mortality in hypertension, there is no study showing that the combination has an additive effect in this regard. Importantly, the ACCOMPLISH study reported that an ACE inhibitor/HCTZ combination was significantly less effective in reducing morbidity and mortality than a combination of the same ACE inhibitor (benazepril) with amlodipine. Since BP was reduced by both fixed combinations to the same extent, either amlodipine confers benefit over and above BP reduction or HCTZ is detrimental over and above BP reduction.

## Direct renin inhibitor and diuretic combinations

What has been said for ACE inhibitors and ARBs in combination with thiazide diuretics holds true as well as direct renin inhibitors. The only one presently available is aliskiren and it comes in a fixed-dose combination with hydrochlorothiazide. Similar to other RAS blockers, presence of hydrochlorothiazide increases the activity of the renin-angiotensin system and makes the blood pressure more amenable to the effects of direct renin inhibitor. Schmieder et al. showed that aliskiren treatment both as monotherapy and with the optional addition od amlodipine provided significantly greater blood pressure reduction than the respective hydrochlorothiazide regimens [47,48].

## Dual RAS blockers

### ACE inhibitors and ARBs

There are several reasons why the combination of an ACE inhibitor and an ARB should have some additional effects with regard to both BP and hypertensive target organ disease. Indeed, several small studies have demonstrated an additive effect of this combination, not so much on BP, but for microproteinuria and also for hemodynamic features in patients with heart failure. In the Candesartan and Lisinopril Microalbuminuria (CALM) study, for instance, 20 mg of lisinopril was combined with 16 mg of candesartan [49]. This combination led to a further decrease in BP and a further reduction in microproteinuria in patients with diabetes and hypertension. However, we cannot possibly conclude from this and other similar studies that the combination had an additive effect because only relatively small doses of the two drug classes were added to each other. A factorial design study, combining increasing doses of losartan with increasing doses of enalapril in a substantial number of patients, showed no additive effects of the two drugs with regard to BP. In order to show that there was additive efficacy, the upper dose range would have to be explored. The addition of amlodipine to patients taking 80 mg of lisinopril would clearly further lower arterial pressure. In contrast, it has not been demonstrated that the addition of an ARB to patients who take the same dose of an ACE inhibitor would have additional effects on either BP or any other surrogate end point. In the Val-HeFT study, the addition of valsartan to an ACE inhibitor seemed to have an additive effect in certain patients [45]. Again, in this study, the potential of the ACE inhibitor, or the ARB, was not exhausted before the other drug was added. More importantly, in the recent ONgoing Telmisartan Alone and in combination with Ramipril Global Endpoint Trial (ONTARGET), the combination of ramipril with telmisartan showed no benefit, despite a lower BP, when compared with the monotherapeutic arm [50]. In fact, despite the decrease in albuminuria, renal outcome was worse in the combination arm. In summary, there is little reason to combine an ACE inhibitor with an ARB for the treatment of BP per se. However, this combination may have some merit in patients with heart failure and seems to be distinctly beneficial in patients with proteinuria/diabetic renal disease.

### Direct renin inhibitor and an ARB

A modest but significant decrease in BP was observed when aliskiren (300 mg) was added to valsartan (320 mg) in a double-blind study of 1797 patients [51]. A fall in BP with the combination therapy was less than one would have expected by the addition of either a thiazide diuretic or a calcium antagonist. The combination was as well tolerated as aliskiren or valsartan alone. As blockade of the renin–angiotensin cascade by either an ACE inhibitor or an ARB increases plasma renin activity, the argument has been put forward that the addition of a direct renin inhibitor could have additional benefits. At present, no outcome data are available to support this hypothesis. Nevertheless, a randomized, double-blind trial (Aliskiren Trial in Type 2 Diabetes Using Cardio-Renal Endpoints [ALTITUDE]) has been designed to answer this question and is currently in progress [51].

### Calcium antagonists and RAS blockers

Both dihydropyridine and nondihydropyridine calcium antagonists lend themselves to combination with RAS blockers (Figure 16). The fact that this combination is attractive is emphasized by the numerous combinations that have become available in recent years (Figures 17–19). Among the available

| Differences between calcium antagonists | | |
|---|---|---|
| | Dihydropyridine | Nondihydropyridine |
| BP | ++ | ++ |
| Heart rate | − | ↓ |
| Sympathetic activity | ↑ | ↓ |
| Secondary cardiac protection | − | + |
| ↓ Proteinuria | ↓ | ↓↓ |
| Adverse effects | | |
| Pedal edema | ++ | + |
| Constipation | + | ++ |

Figure 16 **Differences between calcium antagonists.** BP, blood pressure; ↑, increase; ↓, decrease; −, no effect.

## Possible synergism resulting from a combination of a calcium antagonist and a RAS blocker

| | DHP calcium | Non-DHP calcium antagonist | RAS blocker |
|---|---|---|---|
| **Kidneys** | | | |
| ↑ Renal blood flow | Yes | Yes | Yes |
| ↑ Efferent vasodilation | Little | Yes | Yes |
| ↑ Afferent vasodilation | Yes | Yes | Yes |
| ↓ Microproteinuria | Little | Yes | Yes |
| ↑ Renoprotection | Unknown | Possible | Yes |
| **Vascular tree** | | | |
| ↓ Endothelin-mediated vasoconstriction | Yes | Yes | No |
| ↑ Nitric oxide release | No | No | Yes |
| ↑ Arterial compliance | Yes | Yes | Yes |
| ↓ Vascular hypertrophy | Yes | Yes | Yes |
| ↓ Atherogenesis | Yes | Yes | Yes |
| **Heart** | | | |
| ↓ Left ventricular hypertrophy | Yes | Yes | Yes |
| ↑ Left ventricular filing | Yes | Yes | Yes |
| ↑ Contractility, unloading | Some | No | Yes |
| ↑ Coronary flow | Yes | Yes | Some |
| Secondary 'cardioprotection' | No | Some | Yes |

Figure 17 **Possible synergism resulting from a combination of a calcium antagonist and a RAS blocker.** ↑, increase; ↓, decrease; ACE, angiotensin-converting enzyme; DHP, dihydropyridine; RAS, renin–angiotensin system. Adapted from Opie & Messerli [52].

## Fixed-dose calcium antagonist and ACE inhibitor combinations

Amlopidine 2.5, 5 or 10 mg/benazepril 10, 20, or 40 mg

Diltiazem 180 mg/enalapril 5 mg

Felodipine 5 mg/enalapril 5 mg

Verapamil 180 or 240 mg/trandolapril 1, 2 or 4 mg

Felodipine 5 mg/ramipril 5 mg

Figure 18 **Fixed-dose calcium antagonist and ACE inhibitor combinations.** ACE, angiotensin-converting inhibitor.

**Fixed-dose calcium antagonist and ARB combinations**

Amlodipine 5 or 10 mg/valsartan 160 or 320 mg

Amlodipine 5 or 10 mg/olmesartan medoxomil 20 or 40 mg

Amlodipine 5 or 10 mg/telmisartan 40 or 80 mg

Figure 19 **Fixed-dose calcium antagonist and ARB combinations.** ARB, angiotensin-receptor blocker.

ACE inhibitor/calcium antagonist combinations, the most important ones are verapamil with trandolapril and amlodipine with benazepril. Both of these combinations have been tested in outcome studies. In INVEST, verapamil with trandolapril was compared to atenolol with HCTZ in over 22,000 patients with hypertension and coronary artery disease [53]. Although there was no difference in primary outcome, the risk of new-onset diabetes was substantially lower in the verapamil plus trandolapril arm than in the atenolol plus HCTZ arm. Similarly, in the 19,000-patient Anglo-Scandinavian Cardiac Outcomes Trial (ASCOT) study, the risk of new-onset diabetes was substantially lower in the amlodipine plus trandolapril arm when compared to the atenolol plus thiazide arm [54]. Moreover, in ACCOMPLISH, patients receiving the amlodipine plus benazepril combination had a 20% greater reduction in morbidity and mortality than those in the benazepril with HCTZ arm. This would indicate that either amlodipine had a benefit over and above BP reduction or that HCTZ was detrimental.

As previously mentioned, ARBs are better tolerated than ACE inhibitors. It is therefore not surprising that several ARB/calcium antagonist fixed-dose combinations have also been approved recently. The first combination to be launched was amlodipine with valsartan, which is now also available in a triple combination with HCTZ. Amlodipine has also been combined with olmesartan and telmisartan. All of these fixed combinations are exceedingly well tolerated and have been shown, to some extent, to reduce the pedal edema associated with amlodipine monotherapy.

In my opinion, the ACCOMPLISH study has relegated thiazides to third-line therapy. The most common combination for a majority of patients in uncomplicated hypertension should be a RAS blocker and a calcium antagonist.

## Synergism of combination therapy

The most common adverse effect of the dihydropyridine calcium antagonist is pedal edema, which is clearly dose dependent. Pedal edema is seen in about 5% of patients on amlodipine 5 mg, in 25% of patients on amlodipine 10 mg, and in over 80% of patients on amlodipine 20 mg (which is above the FDA-approved dose). Pedal edema is predominantly caused by arteriolar dilatation that increases intracapillary pressure (capillary hypertension) and thereby causes fluid exudation into the interstitium (Figure 20).

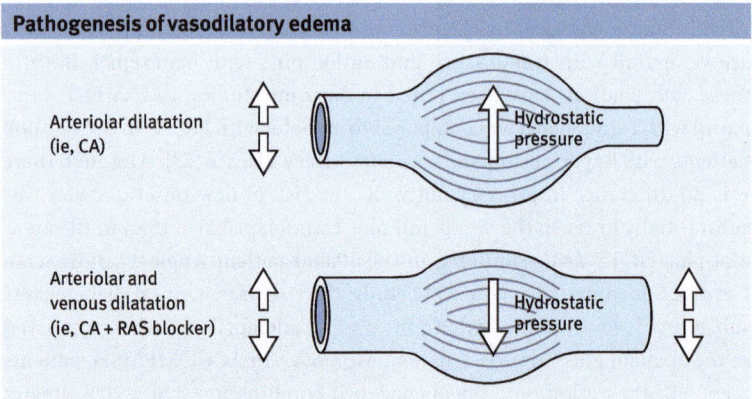

**Figure 20 Pathogenesis of vasodilatory edema.** CA, calcium antagonist; RAS, renin–angiotensin–aldosterone system.

Any drug that causes venular dilatation may diminish capillary hypertension and decrease pedal edema. Both ACE inhibitors and ARBs are known to have this effect. Thus, unsurprisingly, pedal edema was shown to dissipate when benazepril was added to amlodipine in several well-documented studies (Figure 21). In the Lotrel: Gauging Improved Control (LOGIC) trial [55], patients were included on the basis of pedal edema. After 4 weeks, pedal edema diminished significantly in over 80% of patients when they were switched from amlodipine monotherapy to the fixed combination of amlodipine and benazepril (Figure 21) [56,57]. Even with higher doses of amlodipine, such as 20 mg, equally high doses of RAS blockade will diminish pedal edema. Of note, this form of edema is not caused by salt or water retention. Dihydropyridine calcium antagonists have a direct natriuretic effect; therefore, the pedal edema seen with dihydropyridine calcium antagonists does not respond well to diuretic therapy.

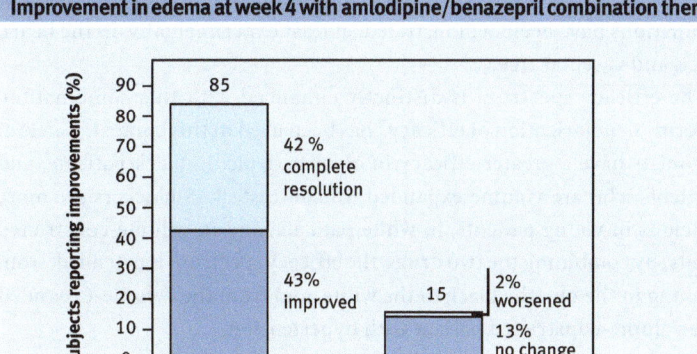

**Figure 21  Improvement in edema at week 4 with amlodipine/benazepril combination therapy.** Blood pressure control but pedal edema with amlodipine (n=1493). Improvement in edema was similar in men and women. Reproduced from Messerli & Grossman [57].

A further advantage of the combination of a dihydropyridine calcium antagonist with an ACE inhibitor is the renoprotective properties (Figure 22).

| Renoprotective properties | |
| --- | --- |
| **Intrarenal effects of RAS blockers** | **Intrarenal effects of calcium antagonists** |
| Reduce intraglomerular pressure | Improve glomerular permeability |
| Improve glomerular permeability | Reduce glomerulosclerosis |
| inhibit glomerular hypertrophy | Reduce formation of oxygen free radicals |
| Prevent glomerulosclerosis | Prevent glomerular hypertrophy |
| Reduce mesangial matrix expansion | Increase natriuresis |
| Reduce interstitial fibrosis | Reduce platelet aggregation |
| Inhibit procollagen formation | Reduce intracellular calcium accumulation |
| Increase natriuresis | reduce renal hypermetabolism |
| Reduce proteinuria | reduce proteinuria |

**Figure 22  Renoprotective properties.** RAS, renin–angiotensin–aldosterone system. Adapted from Opie & Messerli [47].

Although dihydropyridine calcium antagonists are known to reduce micro-proteinuria in patients with diabetes (as was demonstrated in the Syst–Eur study), they are much less efficacious in this regard than RAS blockers. Blockers of the RAS (ie, either ACE inhibitors or ARBs) are the drugs of choice in patients with hypertensive diabetic renal disease. They have been shown, to some extent, to reduce microproteinuria independently of their antihypertensive effect.

Other synergistic effects of the calcium antagonist and RAS blocker combinations have been demonstrated, at least experimentally, in the heart, kidney, and vascular tree.

The efficacy spectrum is distinctly enhanced with this combination. The term "depolarization of efficacy" has been used in this context. Calcium antagonists have a greater efficacy in older patients, in black patients, and in patients who are volume expanded. In contrast, RAS blockers are more efficacious in young patients, in white patients, and in volume-constricted patients. By combining the two drugs, the efficacy spectrum is extended, from the young to the old, the black to the white, and from the volume-expanded to the volume-constricted patient with hypertension.

## Outcome trials

The ASCOT study further attests to the benefit of the combination of an ACE inhibitor with a dihydropyridine calcium antagonist [54]. ASCOT was designed to compare the effect of the standard antihypertensive regimen (a beta-blocker and a diuretic) with that of a more contemporary regimen (calcium antagonist and an ACE inhibitor) on coronary artery disease.

A total of almost 20,000 patients were randomized to either atenolol plus bendroflumethiazide (if needed) or amlodipine plus perindopril (if needed). The trial was interrupted prematurely because of distinct benefits in the amlodipine/perindopril arm. Specifically, compared with atenolol/ thiazide, amlodipine/perindopril resulted in a significant reduction in all-cause mortality and coronary events of about 15%, a reduction in fatal and nonfatal stroke of 25%, a reduction in cardiovascular mortality of 25%, and an impressive reduction in new-onset diabetes of 30% (Figure 23).

Although BP with amlodipine/perindopril was lowered by a further 2.9/1.8 mmHg than with atenolol/bendroflumethiazide, it seems unlikely that this small decrease in BP would account for the impressive benefits.

In the randomized, double-blind Avoiding Cardiovascular events through Combination therapy in Patients Living with Systolic Hypertension (ACCOMPLISH) trial, 11,506 patients with hypertension who were at high risk for cardiovascular events were randomized to either benazepril plus amlodipine or benazepril plus HCTZ [57]. The study was terminated early because there was a significant 20% reduction in primary outcome events (cardiovascular death, nonfatal MI, nonfatal stroke, hospitalization for angina, resuscitation after sudden cardiac arrest, and coronary revascularization) in the benazepril/amlodipine arm when compared with the benazepril/HCTZ arm. The authors concluded that, in this population, the benazepril/amlodipine

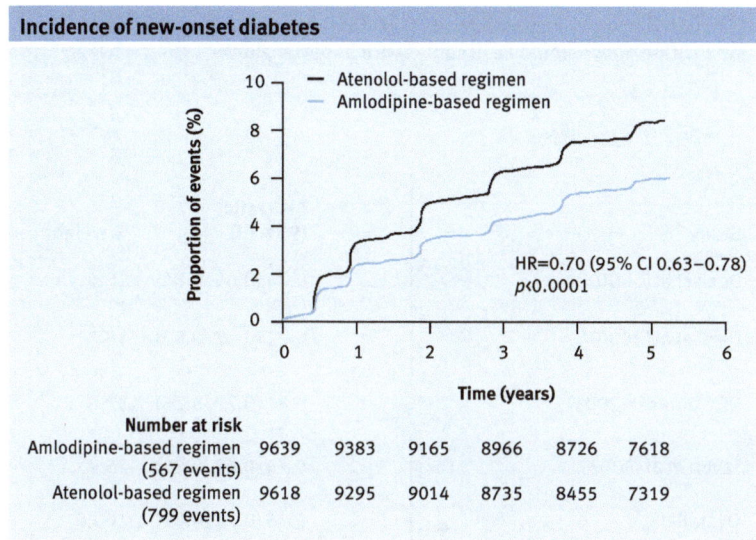

**Incidence of new-onset diabetes**

HR=0.70 (95% CI 0.63–0.78)
p<0.0001

| Number at risk | | | | | | |
|---|---|---|---|---|---|---|
| Amlodipine-based regimen (567 events) | 9639 | 9383 | 9165 | 8966 | 8726 | 7618 |
| Atenolol-based regimen (799 events) | 9618 | 9295 | 9014 | 8735 | 8455 | 7319 |

**Figure 23 Incidence of new-onset diabetes.** HR, hazard ratio. Reproduced with permission from Dahlof et al. [54].

combination was superior to the benazepril/HCTZ combination in reducing cardiovascular events. BP was lowered to the same extent in both combination arms. Of note, many patients in the ACCOMPLISH trial had previous coronary artery disease and diabetes and perhaps, therefore, do not fully represent the broad population of patients with hypertension. Nevertheless, it seems that RAS blockade plus amlodipine confers more benefits than does RAS blockade plus HCTZ.

## Pill burden and compliance

Experienced clinicians have long recognized that the patient's compliance with a given treatment regimen depends, to some extent, on its complexity. As a simple rule, the more pills a patient has to take the sicker he or she feels and the lesser the compliance. This is particularly true when the treatment regimen requires dosing several times a day. Fixed combinations, therefore, have a distinct advantage. Putting two or three drugs into the same pill may reduce side effects; thus, the patient feels less sick and compliance may be enhanced. Indeed, a meta-analysis of four hypertension studies documented a 24% decreased risk of medication noncompliance with a fixed-drug combination regimen when compared with the same medications taken in two separate pills (Figure 24) [58].

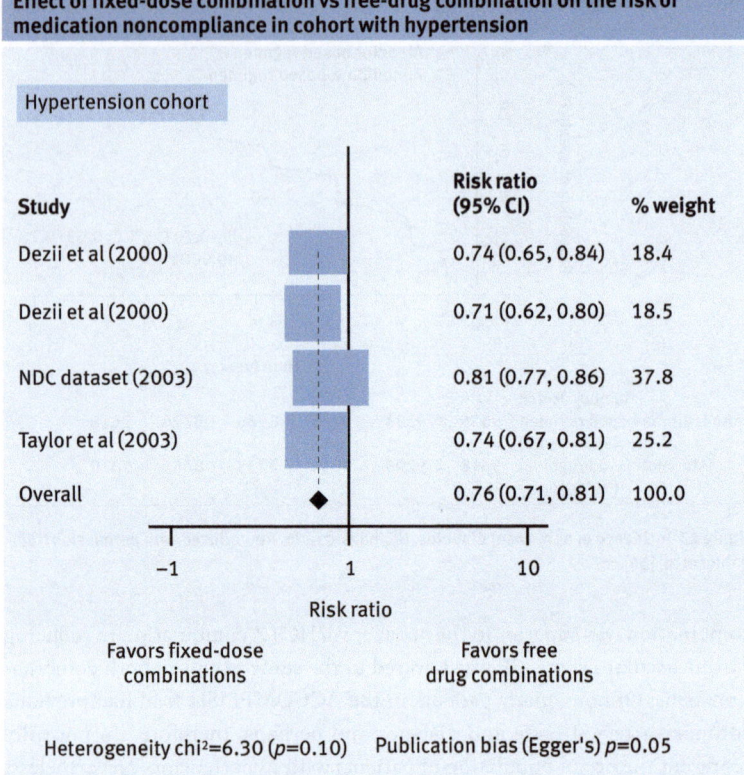

**Figure 24 Effect of fixed-dose combination vs free-drug combination on the risk of medication noncompliance in cohort with hypertension.** Vertical solid line = null effect; vertical dotted line = overall effect on compliance; boxes and horizontal lines = relative risk (95% CI). Reproduced with permission from Bangalore et al. [58].

## When not to use fixed combination therapy

As attractive as fixed combinations are, and although many patients benefit from them, it should be remembered that not every patient with mild to moderately severe hypertension is a candidate for such therapy. Patients need to be thoroughly informed that they are taking a combination of drugs, such as an ARB and a diuretic, in the same pill. Commonly, the labeling of fixed combinations may be deceptive to patients and physicians. In numerous instances, patients have been given inappropriate medication because the physician was not familiar with the ingredients of a fixed combination or the patient did not reveal to the physician that they were taking a fixed combination.

Occasionally, some therapeutic flexibility is lost when a patient is taking a fixed combination drug, and this could be a disadvantage in certain clinical situations. For instance, the need for diuresis may vary a great deal depending on the dietary salt intake. This is particularly true in disease states that are susceptible to sudden unexpected changes such as heart failure or severe coronary artery disease. However, even in patients who appear hemodynamically stable, prolonged aerobic exercise may lead to fluid volume depletion and, thereby, eliminate the need for the diuretic therapy that is part of the fixed combination. In situations like this, it may be preferable to steer clear of a fixed combination and allow the patient some self-medication. However, patients who are able, and willing, to adjust their medications according to daily activity are exceedingly rare. In the great majority of patients with uncomplicated hypertension, fixed combination therapy will lower BP with comfort and convenience.

# Chapter 11

# Comorbid conditions

## Metabolic syndrome and new-onset diabetes

The prevalence of obesity, the metabolic syndrome, and frank diabetes has doubled in the USA over the past decade. With more than 60% of adults and 30% of children classified as overweight or obese, the USA has become the fattest nation on earth. Approximately half of all overweight individuals have insulin resistance and 25% of the population of the USA has multiple risk factors for cardiovascular disease. Cardiovascular risk factors tend to cluster, and insulin resistance or diabetes, obesity, and hypertension are common in the same patient. Ever since the pioneering observation of Colin Dollery's team [59,60] more than 20 years ago, a variety of studies have documented that long-term diuretic therapy, particularly when combined with a beta-blocker, diminishes glucose tolerance and increases the risk of new-onset diabetes. Conversely, as has been revealed in more recent trials, treatment with antihypertensive drugs, such as blockers of the RAS or calcium antagonists, appears to decrease this risk (Figure 25).

### The ALPINE study

The recent Antihypertensive Treatment and Lipid Profile in a North of Sweden Efficacy Evaluation (ALPINE) study was designed to compare the effects of antihypertensive therapy on glucose metabolism in almost 400 patients with uncomplicated hypertension who had never been treated [62]. Patients were randomized to either an ARB (with addition of calcium antagonist, if needed) or a thiazide diuretic (and a beta-blocker, if needed). After only 1 year of follow-up, 18 patients in the diuretic arm reached diagnostic criteria of the metabolic syndrome and nine had developed frank diabetes. The corresponding numbers in the ARB arm were five and one, respectively.

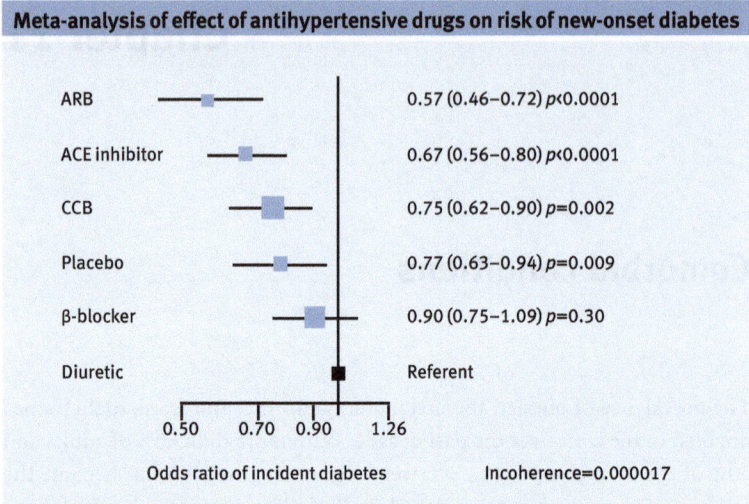

**Figure 25  Meta-analysis of effect of antihypertensive drugs on risk of new-onset diabetes.** Results of network meta-analysis of 22 clinical trials. Trials included 143,153 patients. Initial diuretic used as referent agent. Size of squares (representing the point estimate for each class of antihypertensive drugs) is proportional to number of patients who developed incident diabetes. Horizontal lines indicate 95% confidence interval (CI). Odds ratios to the left of the vertical line at unity denote a protective effect (compared with initial diuretic). Individual pair-wise comparisons between diuretic vs beta-blocker ($p$=0.30), placebo vs calcium channel blocker (CCB) ($p$=0.72), angiotensin-converting enzyme (ACE) inhibitor vs angiotensin receptor blocker (ARB) ($p$=0.16) did not achieve significance ($p$<0.05). Reproduced with permission from Elliott [61].

## The VALUE study

In the VALUE study, more than 15,000 patients with hypertension and one or more additional risk factor were randomized to either amlodipine or valsartan [32].

Investigators found that new-onset diabetes was 23% less common in the patients treated with valsartan than in those treated with amlodipine, despite the fact that BP control was significantly better with amlodipine throughout the study. These results have to be interpreted in the context of the ALLHAT study [43], in which the risk of new-onset diabetes was significantly lower with amlodipine than with chlorthalidone, but not as low as with lisinopril. Of note, however, patients who were randomized to amlodipine had significantly greater hypokalemia than patients who were randomized to valsartan. Hypokalemia can impair glucose tolerance by interfering with insulin release from the pancreas. Such a sequence of events was originally proposed by Conn [63] to explain the high risk of diabetes in patients with primary aldosteronism. These findings were subsequently confirmed by the same group in patients with islet cell tumors. Helderman *et al.* [64] reported that glucose intolerance associated with thiazide diuretics could be entirely avoided if whole-body potassium balance was maintained. Thus, the higher risk of de novo diabetes in the amlodipine arm could possibly be explained by the greater prevalence of hypokalemia.

## The ALLHAT trial

In the ALLHAT study [43], about 10% of the total study population of patients developed new-onset diabetes during the 4- to 6-year duration of the study. Of note, the risk of becoming diabetic was between 40% and 65% higher in patients on chlorthalidone-based therapy than in patients on lisinopril-based therapy, and between 18% and 30% higher in patients on chlorthalidone than in those on amlodipine.

The ALLHAT investigators [43] reassuringly state that, *"Overall, these metabolic differences did not translate into more cardiovascular events or into higher all-cause mortality in the chlorthalidone group."* That this statement was used almost verbatim by the authors of the JNC 7 report [2] is perhaps not surprising given that more than half of them were ALLHAT investigators. However, these reassuring words may strike the practicing physician as slightly myopic given that the follow-up in ALLHAT after the diagnosis of diabetes was 2–4 years. Antihypertensive therapy is most often lifelong and a follow-up lasting a few years is unlikely to give us any information as to the cardiovascular morbidity and mortality related to thiazide diuretic-associated diabetes.

## Long-term follow-up

The recent thorough study of Verdecchia *et al.* [65] has thrown some light on this issue. The authors report up to 16 years of follow-up of almost 800 initially untreated hypertensive patients, 6.5% of whom had diabetes at the onset, and 5.8% of whom developed new-onset diabetes throughout the study. The fasting blood sugar at entry, as well as diuretic treatment on follow-up, were independent, powerful predictors of new-onset diabetes ($p<0.0001$, and $p<0.004$, respectively). Most importantly, compared with individuals who never developed diabetes, the risk for cardiovascular disease during the follow-up was very similar in patients who developed diabetes (odds ratio [OR] 2.92, 95% confidence interval [CI]: 1.33–6.41; $p=0.007$) and in the group that had pre-existing diabetes (OR 3.57, 95% CI: 1.65–7.73; $p=0.001$). Patients with new-onset diabetes, and those with a prior diagnosis of diabetes, were almost three times as likely to develop subsequent cardiovascular disease than those who remained free of diabetes. These provocative findings not only show, again, that antihypertensive therapy with a thiazide diuretic alone or, if needed, in combination with a beta-blocker confers a substantial risk of new-onset diabetes, but also more importantly that patients who have become diabetic will suffer all the adverse sequelae of this disease. Alderman *et al.* [66], in a study of almost 7000 patients, showed that cardiovascular disease increased in hypertensive diuretic users who developed hyperglycemia even when BP was well controlled. The authors stated, "*Cardiovascular disease incidence has a direct dose–response relation with diuretic used with frequent users having the highest rate*" [66]. Conceivably, the combination of a diuretic and an ACE inhibitor may confer a lesser risk of new-onset diabetes. At least in one small short-term study, ACE inhibitors seemed to prevent the metabolic deleterious effect of the diuretic thiazide [66]. By preventing hypokalemia RAS blockers may lower the risk of diuretic-induced metabolic adverse events.

## Antihypertensive therapy in the diabetic patient

The above considerations make it clear that the patient with diabetes and hypertension benefits from blockade of the RAS more than from any other pharmacologic intervention. Clearly, therefore, blockers of the RAS are a cornerstone in antihypertensive therapy for the diabetic patient. Unfortunately, many patients with diabetes and hypertension are black or have hyporeninemic hypoaldosteronism. In these patient groups, the antihypertensive efficacy of ACE inhibitors and ARBs is blunted. However, despite lowering BP less well, ACE inhibitors, and probably ARBs, still have distinct nephroprotective and possibly cardioprotective effects. Calcium antagonists have been shown to exert impressive morbidity and mortality benefits in the patient with diabetes and hypertension and, therefore, should be added as second-line agents. Dihydropyridine calcium antagonists may lower BP somewhat more than the nondihydropyridines, although the latter are preferred in the diabetic patient because of their synergistic effect on proteinuria when given with an ACE inhibitor. Low-dose thiazide diuretics are acceptable, preferentially as third-line agents. In combination with a RAS blocker, the diabetogenic effect of thiazide diuretics is relatively small. Traditional beta-blockers should be used sparingly in diabetic patients, as these drugs have been shown to increase the risk of diabetes and also to cause systematic weight gain. Of note, carvedilol seems to be void of these effects and, therefore, is the beta-blocker of choice in patients with diabetes.

In patients with diabetes post-MI, the benefits of the beta-blocker clearly outweigh its potential negative effect.

## Cerebrovascular disease

Calcium antagonists have been shown to diminish the risk of stroke somewhat better than other drug classes. In the MRC study, diuretics were shown to have a specific cerebroprotective effect; at any given BP level, the risk of stroke was less in patients treated with a diuretic than in those on placebo [40]. Thus, a patient with manifest cerebrovascular disease should primarily be treated with a diuretic or a calcium antagonist. The jury seems to be out, at present, on the effect of ACE inhibitors; one study showed a solid benefit, whereas others showed no distinct effect [68]. Of note, in the ONTARGET study, no significant difference was seen with regard to stroke prevention between the three treatment arms (ramipril, telmisartan and a combination of the two). There is little question though that ARBs are good drugs for preventing strokes, as was shown in a recent meta-analysis (Figure 26) [68].

## Hypertensive heart disease, coronary artery disease, and heart failure

ACE inhibitors, and possibly ARBs, are the best monotherapeutic way to reduce LVH, followed by calcium antagonists, diuretics, and, distinctly less effective, beta-blockers. ACE inhibitors are also a cornerstone in the management of the patient with heart failure and the post-MI patient. ACE inhibitors, and possibly ARBs, are probably the best choice for initial therapy in the patient with hypertensive heart disease. Beta-blockers have morbidity and mortality benefits in the post-MI patient but do not have any primary cardioprotective effects in hypertension. Low-dose beta-blockade is also very useful in patients with heart failure. As shown in the Val-HeFT study, the combination of an ACE inhibitor and an ARB may benefit certain patients with heart failure [45]. Morbidity and mortality benefits of diuretics have never been documented in heart failure. However, as in any other edematous state, diuretics will bring symptomatic relief. Calcium antagonists are useful in the patient with hypertensive heart disease and stable coronary artery disease. However, calcium antagonists should be avoided in patients with unstable angina and those with heart failure. If a calcium antagonist is needed in a patient with heart failure, amlodipine seems to be the drug of choice. With regard to prevention of coronary artery disease, it seems that ACE inhibitors are more efficacious than are the ARBs, although the significance is borderline (Figure 27) [68].

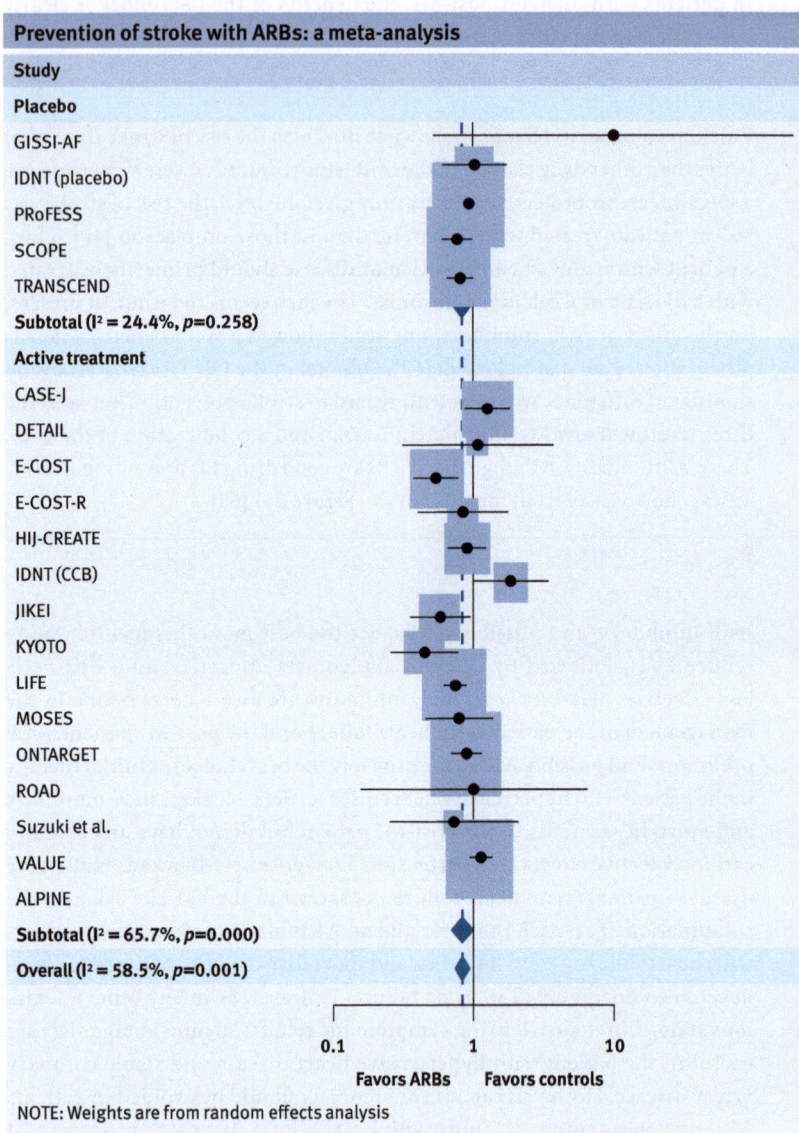

**Prevention of stroke with ARBs: a meta-analysis**

**Figure 26 Prevention of stroke with ARBs: a meta-analysis.** There was a significant reduction in the risk of stroke with angiotensin receptor blockers (ARBs) compared with controls. The size of the markers represents the weight of each trial. Meta-analysis was performed using the search terms 'angiotensin receptor blockers' with the inclusion criteria of being a randomized comparison with follow-up for at least 1 year, enrolling non-heart failure patients and evaluating outcomes of interest. Reproduced with permission from Messerli et al. [68].

| OR (95% CI) | Events, ARBs | Events, control | % Weight |
|---|---|---|---|
| 9.03 (0.49, 167.93) | 4/722 | 0/720 | 0.16 |
| 1.06 (0.61, 1.83) | 28/579 | 26/569 | 3.51 |
| 0.94 (0.85, 1.04) | 880/10,146 | 934/10,186 | 12.28 |
| 0.76 (0.57, 1.01) | 89/2477 | 115/2460 | 7.64 |
| 0.82 (0.64, 1.06) | 112/2954 | 136/2972 | 8.29 |
| **0.89 (078, 1.02)** | **1113/16,878** | **1211/16,907** | **31.90** |
| | | | |
| 1.28 (0.87, 1.88) | 60/2354 | 47/2349 | 5.57 |
| 1.09 (0.34, 3.47) | 6/120 | 6/130 | 0.98 |
| 0.56 (0.38, 0.81) | 47/1053 | 77/995 | 5.79 |
| 0.85 (0.40, 1.80) | 17/69 | 20/72 | 2.12 |
| 0.92 (0.61, 1.39) | 45/1024 | 49/1025 | 5.12 |
| 1.87 (0.99, 3.54) | 28/579 | 15/567 | 2.77 |
| 0.57 (0.35, 0.94) | 25/1541 | 43/1540 | 4.02 |
| 0.44 (0.26, 0.77) | 19/1517 | 42/1514 | 3.52 |
| 0.73 (0.62, 0.88) | 232/4605 | 309/4588 | 10.37 |
| 0.84 (0.53, 1.32) | 36/681 | 42/671 | 4.50 |
| 0.91 (0.79, 1.05) | 369/8542 | 405/8576 | 11.17 |
| 1.00 (0.14, 7.18) | 2/180 | 2/180 | 0.36 |
| 0.74 (0.25, 2.18) | 6/183 | 8/183 | 1.12 |
| 1.14 (0.97, 1.35) | 322/7649 | 281/7596 | 10.69 |
| (Excluded) | 0/197 | 0/196 | 0.00 |
| **0.86 (0.72, 1.02)** | **1214/30,294** | **1346/30,182** | **68.10** |
| **0.87 (0.77, 1.98)** | **2327/47,172** | **2557/47,089** | **100.00** |

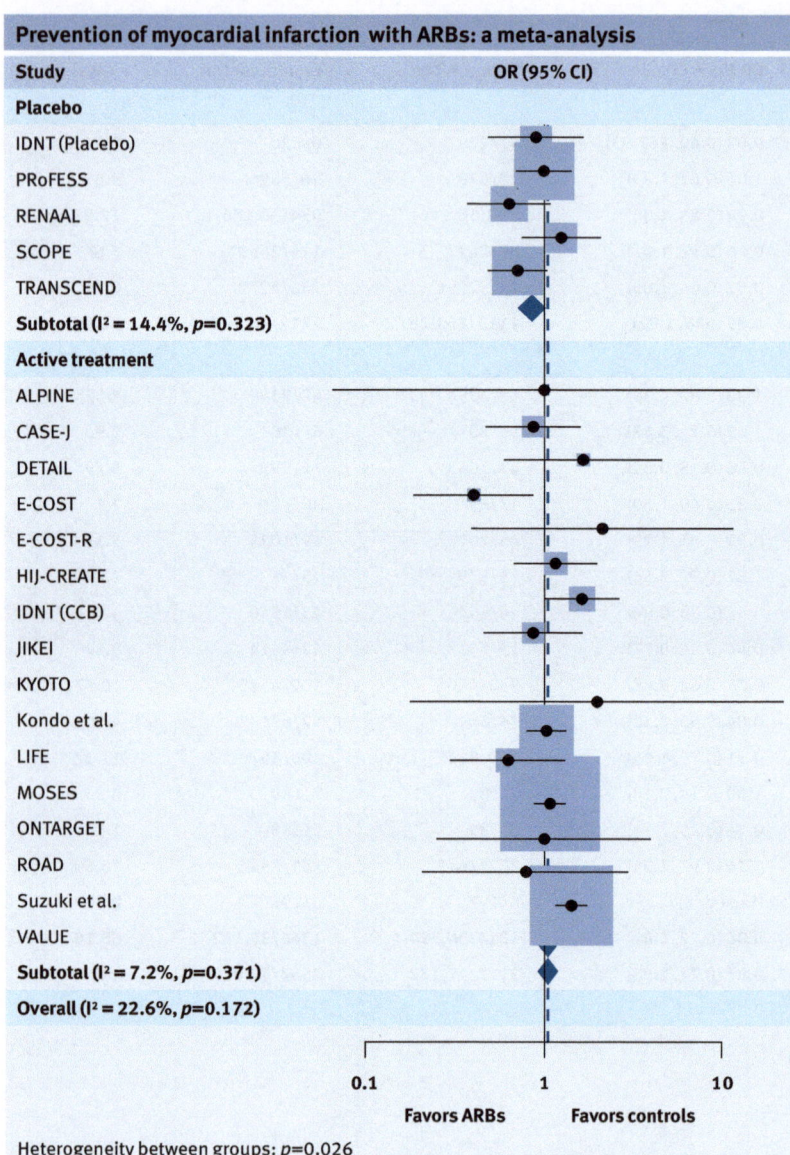

**Figure 27 Prevention of myocardial infarction with ARBs: a meta-analysis.** There was a trend toward increased risk of myocardial infarction with ARBs compared with the active treatment group. The size of the markers represents the weight of each trial. Reproduced with permission from Messerli et al. [68].

| OR (95% CI) | Events, ARBs | Events, control | % Weight |
|---|---|---|---|
| 0.94 (0.61, 1.44) | 44/579 | 46/569 | 2.72 |
| 1.00 (0.80, 1.24) | 168/10,146 | 169/10,186 | 10.88 |
| 0.73 (0.50, 1.06) | 50/751 | 68/762 | 3.50 |
| 1.14 (0.77, 1.70) | 54/2477 | 47/2460 | 3.23 |
| 0.79 (0.61, 1.01) | 116/2954 | 147/2972 | 8.14 |
| **0.90 (0.79, 1.03)** | **432/16,907** | **477/16,949** | **28.48** |
| 0.99 (0.06, 16.02) | 1/197 | 1/196 | 0.07 |
| 0.94 (0.48, 1.83) | 17/2354 | 18/2349 | 1.14 |
| 1.68 (0.58, 4.86) | 9/120 | 6/130 | 0.45 |
| 0.41 (0.19, 0.86) | 10/1053 | 23/995 | 0.90 |
| 2.15 (0.38, 12.16) | 4/69 | 2/72 | 0.17 |
| 1.12 (0.65, 1.92) | 29/1024 | 26/1025 | 1.75 |
| 1.64 (1.00, 2.70) | 44/579 | 27/567 | 2.07 |
| 0.89 (0.46, 1.72) | 17/1541 | 19/1540 | 1.16 |
| 0.63 (0.24, 1.64) | 7/1517 | 11/1514 | 0.56 |
| 2.01 (0.18, 22.34) | 2/203 | 1/203 | 0.09 |
| 1.05 (0.86, 1.29) | 198/4605 | 188/4588 | 12.14 |
| 0.79 (0.51, 1.22) | 39/681 | 48/671 | 2.65 |
| 1.07 (0.94, 1.23) | 440/8542 | 413/8576 | 26.59 |
| 1.00 (0.25, 4.06) | 4/180 | 4/180 | 0.26 |
| 0.80 (0.21, 3.01) | 4/183 | 5/183 | 0.28 |
| 1.18 (1.01, 1.38) | 369/7649 | 313/7596 | 21.26 |
| **1.08 (1.00, 1.18)** | **1194/30,497** | **1105/30,385** | **71.52** |
| **1.03 (0.96, 1.10)** | **1626/47,404** | **1582/47,334** | **100.00** |

## Atrial fibrillation

Atrial fibrillation is an under-recognized complication of long-standing hypertension and increases the likelihood of morbidity and mortality – at least doubling the risk for cardiovascular death or stroke. The main factors predicting development of atrial fibrillation are age, male sex, severity of hypertension, obesity, and presence of LVH on electrocardiogram. Some findings suggest that the choice of BP-lowering treatment could reduce the risk of developing atrial fibrillation. Notably, treatment that inhibits the RAS might be more likely to prevent new-onset atrial fibrillation than other antihypertensitive drug classes. The mechanism for this benefit is unclear but could be, at least in part, dependent on favorable structural regression of left ventricular mass and a reduction in left atrial size.

## Hyperlipidemia

Diuretics and traditional beta-blockers, such as atenolol and metoprolol, are known to increase triglycerides and to lower high-density lipoprotein cholesterol levels (Figure 28). In contrast, vasodilating beta-blockers, such as carvedilol, and ACE inhibitors, calcium antagonists, and alpha-blockers are metabolically neutral, or may even have a slightly favorable effect on lipoproteins.

| The effects of antihypertensive agents on lipids | | | |
| --- | --- | --- | --- |
| Antihypertensive agent | TC | TG | HDL |
| Diuretics (dose dependent) | ↑ 3–11% | ↑ –10–20% | NC |
| Central alpha agonists | NC | ? | NC |
| Ganglionic blockers | ? | ? | ? |
| Peripheral alpha antagonists | ↓ 4% | ↓ 8% | ↑ 4% |
| Beta-blockers | ↑ 0–5% | ↑ 8–25% | ↓ 5–20% |
|   Carvedilol | NC | NC | NC |
|   Nebivolol | NC | NC | NC |
| RAS blockers | NC | NC | NC |
| Calcium antagonists | NC | NC | NC |
| Hydralazine, minoxidil | (rarely given alone; effects not known) | | |

Figure 28 **The effects of antihypertensive agents on lipids.** ↑, increase; ↓, decrease; ?, uncertain; ACE, angiotensin-converting inhibitor; HDL, high-density lipoprotein component; NC, no change; TC, total cholesterol; TG, triglyceride. Adapted from Cohn et al. [45].

## Dementia

Dementia is a major concern in the elderly hypertensive patient. Patients with hypertension have been shown to suffer cognitive dysfunction and dementia of all types more commonly than do normotensive subjects. The effects of antihypertensive therapy on dementia are not well documented. However, provocative findings from the Syst–Eur trial have shown that dihydropyridine calcium antagonists reduce dementia by as much as 55% (Figure 29) [69]. In some, but not all, studies, statins also showed a beneficial effect on dementia. Although this remains to be confirmed, it nevertheless makes calcium antagonists, possibly in combination with a statin, an attractive choice for the elderly patient. More recently ARBs and lipophilic ACE inhibitors have also been reported to reduce the risk of dementia.

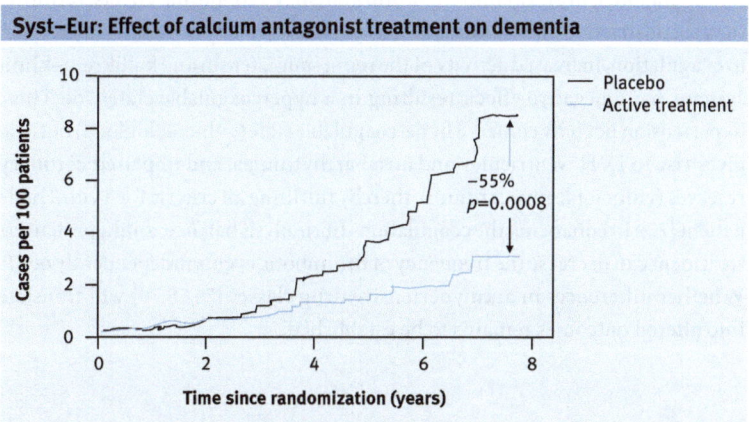

**Syst–Eur: Effect of calcium antagonist treatment on dementia**

Figure 29 **Syst–Eur: Effect of calcium antagonist treatment on dementia.** Syst–Eur, Systolic Hypertension in Europe. Reproduced from Forette et al. [69].

## The prothrombotic paradox

Hypertension by definition is a hemodynamic disorder and, as such, exposes the arterial tree to increased pulsatile stress. Paradoxically, however, most major complications of longstanding hypertension (ie, heart attack and strokes) are thrombotic rather than hemorrhagic, referred to as the so-called thrombotic paradox of hypertension. Virchow suggested three components facilitating thrombus formation (Virchow's triad):

- damage to the vessel wall;
- hypercoagulability; and
- abnormal blood flow.

For thromboembolic events to take place, all the components of Virchow's triad must be fulfilled [70]. In hypertensive individuals, abnormalities in blood flow have been well recognized. Hypertension has also been associated with endothelial damage or dysfunction [71] and a hypercoagulable state [70]. This prothrombotic state could be the result of chronic low-grade inflammation. Chronic shear stress can lead to remodeling of the vascular endothelium, turning it from an anticoagulant into a procoagulant surface. The mechanisms leading to endothelial dysfunction are multifactorial and include decreased activity of vasodilator agents [72–74] and increased activity (or sensitivity) to vasoconstrictor agents [73–75]. Overall, fibrinolytic activity is ascertained by the balance between tissue plasminogen activator and plasminogen activator inhibitor type 1 (SERPINE1). With respect to endothelial function, enhanced activity of the renin–angiotensin and kallikrein–kinin systems has opposing effects, resulting in vasoconstriction and vasodilation, respectively [76]. By contrast, with respect to coagulation, increased activity of the renin–angiotensin and kallikrein–kinin systems has a negative effect, resulting in a hypercoagulable state [76]. Thus, hypertension not only confers a hypercoagulable state (vulnerable blood) but also gives rise to LVH, ventricular and atrial arrhythmias, and impaired coronary reserves (vulnerable myocardium), thereby fulfilling all criteria for a vulnerable patient [77]. In enhancing the coagulation–fibrinolysis balance, antihypertensive treatment can decrease the frequency of thrombotic events independently of BP. Whether differences in antihypertensive drug classes [76,78,79] will translate into altered outcomes remains to be established.

# Chapter 12

## Therapeutic challenges

### Nephroprotection

In the patient with diabetic hypertensive renal disease, blockade of the RAS has been shown to be nephroprotective; that is, to diminish proteinuria and slow down the decline in renal function. In type 1 diabetes, most proteinuria studies have used ACE inhibitors, whereas, for type 2 diabetes, ARBs have mostly been used. However, the American Diabetes Association (ADA) have concluded that the evidence was sufficient to state that both drug classes, ACE inhibitors and ARBs, are indicated for nephroprotection in susceptible patients. Although neither ACE inhibitors nor ARBs are labeled for use to decrease proteinuria/albuminuria or to exert any nephroprotective effect, some studies show that nondihydropyridine calcium antagonists, such as diltiazem and verapamil, reduce urinary protein excretion more than the dihydropyridines, specifically nifedipine. A systematic review by Bakris et al. showed a significantly greater reduction of proteinuria with the nondihydropyridine derivatives than with the dihydropyridines in patients with hypertension, regardless of whether or not they had diabetes [80]. However, we should not forget that albuminuria/proteinuria is a surrogate end point that is not synonymous with renal disease. In the ONTARGET study [7], dual RAS blockade diminished albuminuria more than did monotherapy, but renal end points were significantly more common. This would indicate that albuminuria/ proteinuria is not an ironclad surrogate end point for renal outcome.

### Early morning hypertension

Ever since the pioneering studies of Sir George Pickering, we have known that BP follows a distinct diurnal pattern, decreasing throughout the evening to a nadir at midnight, followed by an early morning rise shortly before awakening. This pattern is qualitatively similar in both normotensive and hypertensive patients. Hypertensive complications, such as stroke, acute MI, and sudden death follow a very similar pattern: the time period between 6:00 a.m. and 10:00 a.m. seems to confer the highest risk for these events. In a meta-analysis of

31 studies, Elliott showed a 49% higher stroke risk in the period from 6:00 a.m. to noon than in the remaining hours of the day [81]. Similarly, Kario *et al.* [82] showed a higher prevalence of silent cerebral ischemia and stroke in patients who have a morning surge of BP, as opposed to patients who did not exhibit such a surge. Although the exact relationship between BP and the occurrence of these events remains to be elucidated, good BP control during the critical hours is desirable. Unfortunately, as most antihypertensive drugs are taken in the morning, their antihypertensive efficacy is weakest (at trough) during this critical time period. Recently, some antihypertensive drugs have been redesigned to provide better morning BP control when taken in the evening. Such a chronotherapeutic approach has been documented with long-acting diltiazem and some verapamil formulations. However, it is not yet known whether such a chronotherapeutic approach will improve morbidity and mortality compared with a nonchronotherapeutic approach of the same medication.

## White-coat hypertension and masked hypertension

BP is a very labile hemodynamic parameter; it varies from heartbeat to heartbeat, from morning to evening, from winter to summer, from sleeping to awake, and from sitting to standing. The same holds true for any other cardiovascular hemodynamic parameter, such as heart rate, cardiac output, ejection fraction, or pulmonary wedge pressure. However, the information that is based on invasively obtained measurements is often considered more reliable than information based on simple BP recording. Numerous studies have documented that BP carefully measured by cuff, under standardized conditions in physicians' offices, is a powerful and reliable predictor of morbidity and mortality. More recent studies have documented that 24-hour ambulatory BP monitoring is an even closer surrogate end point for heart attack and stroke than is office-measured BP. As the correlation between 24-hour ambulatory BP measurement and office BP measurement is moderate at best, there will be, not unexpectedly, a significant number of people who are truly hypertensive but in whom the diagnosis is missed by office BP measurements (*masked hypertension*). Conversely, BP may be elevated in the office but not on ambulatory BP monitoring – an entity known to most clinicians as *white-coat hypertension*.

White-coat hypertension is a well-known clinical entity familiar to most physicians. A variety of studies, has shown that the risk of patients with white-coat hypertension is somewhat elevated but distinctly lower than in patients who have sustained hypertension. Despite being common, little is known about how to best manage white-coat hypertension. Out of fear of overtreatment, some physicians are taking a "wait and see" approach in patients. Conversely, out of fear of litigation, some physicians may take an overaggressive therapeutic approach, which can result in hypotension and orthostatic symptoms.

In contrast, masked hypertension is a much less well-known (but not necessarily a less common) entity, which seems to carry a distinctly more serious prognosis. The same entity has been described occasionally as *reversed white-coat hypertension*. It was initially regarded as being rare but was more recently found to be present, to some extent, in about one-third of the hypertensive population. Risk factors for masked hypertension are alcohol, tobacco, and caffeine, as well as physical inactivity. In the PAMELA (Pressioni Arteriose Monitorate E Loro Associazioni) population, patients with masked hypertension had a prevalence of echocardiographic LVH that was much greater than that of normotensive subjects. Inappropriate target organ disease (ie, inappropriate for office BP levels) should therefore trigger a suspicion of masked hypertension and motivate physicians to expose a susceptible patient to 24-hour ambulatory BP monitoring [83].

In the same PAMELA study, it was reported that more than 50% of patients with white-coat or masked hypertension developed sustained hypertension over a 10-year period, and, when compared with normotensives, white coat hypertensives had a 2.5-fold increased risk and masked hypertensives a 1.8-fold increase risk of developing sustained hypertension (Figure 30) [83]. This clearly shows that neither of the two conditions should be shrugged off as innocent observations. Both white-coat hypertension and masked hypertension need to be identified and diagnosed and deserve to be monitored carefully [84].

The clinician should remember that it's much easier to suspect a diagnosis of white-coat hypertension, as patients will usually say that their BP is normal at home. In contrast, masked hypertension needs to be looked out for, and there are only a few clinical hints as to its presence. A normal BP in the clinical setting does not mean that a patient is not at risk from an elevated BP, which can occur at other times of the day. This is particularly true in patients who are treated with antihypertensive drugs that do not cover a full 24-hour period. As the patient takes the medication in the morning, BP values in the physician's office are, most often, normal but may be substantially elevated at the end of the dosing interval (ie, during the night and early morning hours). Thus, in many hypertensive patients, clinic BP is seemingly well controlled, but early morning BP, before taking the medication, may be elevated, thereby accelerating the risk of cardiovascular events. For many clinicians, masked hypertension has unfortunately become a blind spot in antihypertensive therapy. Although a sweeping recommendation that all patients with high BP (or normal BP) should undergo 24-hour ambulatory BP monitoring cannot be made, the presence of inappropriate target organ disease, such as LVH or microalbuminuria, should arise suspicion of masked hypertension and motivate physicians to initiate a further work-up. **With regard to the therapeutic approach, we should remember that white-coat hypertension has a benign prognosis and can only be over-treated; therefore, a conservative approach is probably justified. In contrast, masked hypertension has a much more serious**

**Percentage of patients progressing to and regressing from true hypertension over 10 years**

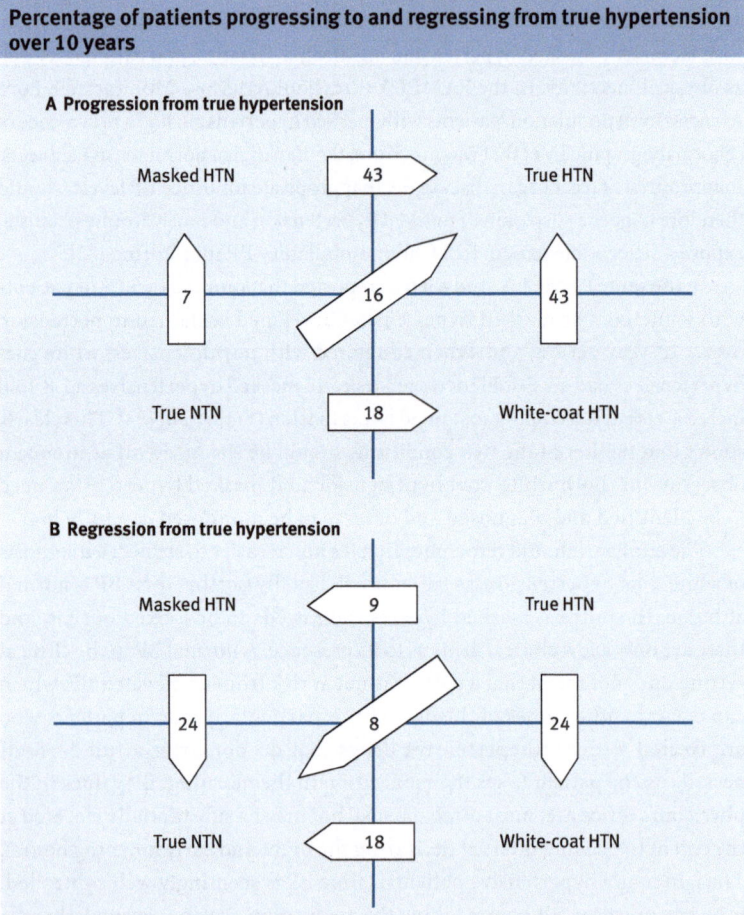

**Figure 30 Percentage of patients progressing and regressing to true hypertension over 10 years.** A, Progression toward true hypertension. Numbers in the figure show the percentage of the patients who progressed toward true hypertension from masked hypertension, true normotension, and white-coat hypertension. NTN indicates normotension; HTN, hypertension. B, Regression from true hypertension. Numbers in the figure show the percentage of the patients who regressed from true hypertension to masked hypertension, true normotension, and white-coat hypertension. Reproduced with permission from Messerli and Makani [84].

**prognosis and can only be under-treated; it deserves, therefore, a thorough evaluation and a more aggressive therapeutic approach.**

## Black patients

Hypertension is more common in black than in white patients, and its course is distinctly more severe. Black patients have a three-times higher mortality rate from cardiovascular disease than do white patients, and their risk of end-stage renal disease is several times greater. These simple facts indicate that cardiovascular diseases, such as hypertension, hyperlipidemia, and diabetes, should be treated most aggressively in the black population. However, the impediments to aggressive therapy in this population are numerous and range from relative inefficacy of certain antihypertensive drug classes and ill-perceived adverse effects, to socioeconomic factors. No racial difference in antihypertensive efficacy has been documented for calcium antagonists and diuretics. In a meta-analysis, calcium antagonists were the only drug class showing efficacy in all BP strata [85]. In contrast, ACE inhibitors and ARBs, at a given dose, have distinctly less effect on BP in black patients than in white patients. The same seems to hold true for heart failure, but not for renal disease. For the same fall in BP, black patients experienced more nephroprotection with an ACE inhibitor than with a calcium antagonist, as demonstrated in the African-American Study of Kidney Disease and Hypertension (AASK) [86].

Importantly, the most dreaded, albeit rare, adverse effect of ACE inhibitor, namely angioedema, is several times more common in black than in white patients. Angioedema can occur after weeks or months of ACE inhibitor therapy and may account for several hundred fatalities per year worldwide. A report from one coroner's office highlights the concerns; it documents that six black patients died of asphyxiation secondary to angioedema of the tongue associated with ACE inhibitor therapy over a period of 3 years [87]. Once solid studies are published attesting to the similar (or, hopefully, even better) outcomes with ARBs in black patients, ACE inhibitors should be avoided all together. The only good news, with regard to the treatment of hypertension in black patients, is that high doses of most antihypertensive drug classes are well tolerated. However, in general, the plateau of the dose–response curve in the black patient is often only reached at a higher dose level than in a white patient.

## Alcohol abuse

The pathogenesis of BP elevation in patients who abuse alcohol is multi-factorial. Acutely, alcohol is a vasodilator but, chronically, it has a direct vasculotoxic effect and produces constriction of vascular smooth muscle.

It stimulates the sympathetic nervous system, as well as the RAS, and may cause thirst and dehydration, which often are counteracted by excessive salt and water retention. Chronic alcohol abuse is not an uncommon cause of seemingly refractory hypertension. Calcium antagonists are the most efficient first-line therapy in the alcoholic hypertensive patient. If combination therapy is needed, a beta-blocker could be useful because it diminishes the activity of the sympathetic nervous system. ACE inhibitors are somewhat less efficacious because of alcohol-associated fluctuations in fluid volume state. Diuretics are often relatively contraindicated because they may trigger an attack of gout in susceptible patients. Not uncommonly, allopuritol or febroxustat may have given to control hyperuricemix before diuretic therapy can be initiated.

Although one or two drinks per day (particularly red wine) may have a beneficial effect on overall cardiovascular risk, as alcohol elevates high-density lipoprotein cholesterol, any higher daily alcohol intake has a detrimental effect on the cardiovascular system. Excessive alcohol intake is a particularly powerful risk factor for hemorrhagic stroke.

## Erectile and orgasmic dysfunction

Long-standing, untreated hypertension is well known to have a negative impact on sexual function and can lead to complete impotence. Unfortunately, antihypertensive drugs still have a bad reputation with regard to erectile function. Some of the older antihypertensive drugs, such as resurpine and guanethidine, have a well-known negative effect on erectile and orgasmic function. Diuretics, beta-blockers, and antiadrenergic drugs, as well as alpha-blockers, diminish erectile function. Failure to ejaculate, or even retrograde ejaculation into the bladder, may occur with some antiadrenergic drugs. In women, diuretics and certain antiadrenergic drugs may interfere with lubrication. Beta-blockers are known to cause orgasmic dysfunction in women and men alike.

BP lowering (by any drug) may by itself, at least initially, have a slight negative impact on erectile function. However, the body fairly rapidly adjusts to the lower BP level and, with modern antihypertensive therapy (calcium antagonists, ACE inhibitors and ARBs), no lasting sexual dysfunction has been reported. On the contrary, in a recent study, the frequency of sexual intercourse actually increased in patients in whom BP was lowered with an ARB when compared with those whose hypertension was left untreated on placebo [88]. This illustrates that low-grade sexual dysfunction, associated with untreated hypertension, can be unmasked by modern antihypertensive therapy.

Sildenafil and its derivatives seem to be safe in patients with hypertension, even if they are being treated with two or more antihypertensive drugs. It should be remembered that sildenafil is a vasodilator and, in general, causes a mild transient decrease in BP. The patient should be warned that the use of sildenafil, in combination with certain antihypertensive drugs, particularly alpha-blockers, could lead to orthostatic symptoms.

## Resistant hypertension

Resistant hypertension is said to be present if, despite triple therapy including a thiazide diuretic, BP remains distinctly above target range. Figure 31 lists some of the more common underlying causes of resistant hypertension. Of particular concern are NSAIDs, as well as the cyclooxygenase 2 (COX2) inhibitors. These drugs elevate BP by a variety of mechanisms, ranging from direct binding with mineralocorticoid receptors to interference with prostaglandin synthetase.

### Some mechanisms of resistance to drug therapy

Nonadherence to therapy

Drug related
- Inappropriate combinations
- Short duration of action

Effects of concomitant therpay
- Sympathomimetics
- Appetite suppressants
- SSRIs, tricyclic antidepressants
- Adrenal steroids (also topical)
- COX2 inhibitors, NSAIDs
- Nasal decongestants
- Oral contraceptives
- Licorice abuse

Associated conditions
- increasing obesity
- Alcohol abuse
- Tobacco abuse
- Abuse of other recreational drugs
- Hyperlipidemia
- Renal insufficiency
- Renovascular hypertension
- Malignant or accelerated hypertension
- Other causes of hypertension

Volume overload
- Inadequate diuretic therapy
- Excess sodium intake
- Fluid retention caused by antihypertensives (pseudoresistance)

Figure 31 **Some mechanisms of resistance to drug therapy.** COX, cyclooxygenase; NSAIDs, nonsteroidal anti-inflammatory drugs; SSRI, selective serotonin reuptake inhibitors.

Very often, the antihypertensive efficacy of ACE inhibitors and ARBs is completely abolished when NSAIDs, or COX2 inhibitors, are added to the regimen. In contrast, these drugs have little, if any, effect on the antihypertensive efficacy of calcium antagonists. Perhaps the most common error is to diagnose resistant hypertension when triple antihypertensive therapy is given without a diuretic. In volume-expanded patients, in those who abuse salt, and in black patients, the antihypertensive efficacy of ACE inhibitors and beta-blockers is blunted. The addition of a diuretic not only diminishes fluid volume retention, but also stimulates the RAS, and makes BP more amenable to the effects of the ACE inhibitor or the ARB. A whole host of other chemical substances, including licorice, topical steroids, and alcohol, can cause resistant hypertension. Therapy with modern oral contraceptives is an unusual reason for resistant hypertension, as estrogen doses have become distinctly lower than in the past. In general, a thorough history and a careful review of all drugs will allow the physician to identify the reason for so-called resistant hypertension. Of note, the most common cause of this entity remains noncompliance with the antihypertensive regimen. Some hints on how to deal with noncompliant patients are outlined in Figure 32.

**Methods of improving compliance**

- Educate the patient about the reason for the medications and their proper use
- Improve patient's social support network (ie, involve spouse or caregiver
- Increase patient's autonomy and involvement in decision making (when appropriate), including home blood pressure monitoring
- Remove barriers to compliance will pill taking (eg, by avoiding large or bad-tasting pills)
- Use cost-saving strategies such as "halfable" pills
- Simplify the therapeutic regimen (minimize the number of pills, frequency of pill taking and the inconvenience of pill taking)
- Integrate pill taking into activities of daily living (eg, shaving, brushing teeth)
- Provide a positive attitude and reinforcement about achieving therapeutic goals

**Figure 32 Methods of improving compliance.** Reproduced from Kaplan [89].

An implantable device that lowers BP by baroreflex stimulation in patients with resistant hypertension is currently in development [89].

## Isolated systolic hypertension

There are three main reasons why isolated systolic hypertension has become increasingly important over the past few years:

- We are seeing more and more elderly patients, and isolated systolic hypertension is the most common form of high BP in the geriatric population.
- Systolic BP has finally been recognized as the most powerful predictor of cardiovascular morbidity and mortality and, therefore, treatment of systolic BP has become more important than that of diastolic BP.
- The treatment goals of systolic BP have become increasingly lower over the past few years, thereby creating numerous hypertensive patients who, according to previous criteria, would not have fulfilled this definition.

Even in very elderly patients, a systolic BP goal of less than 140 mmHg can be a realistic goal with modern antihypertensive therapy, although sometimes there will have to be a compromise between the BP goal and the patient's well-being, health plan, and wallet.

The most common pitfall encountered in the treatment of isolated systolic hypertension is the failure to recognize that bradycardia can be its major perpetrator. Any decrease in heart rate is prone to an increase in stroke volume; a higher stroke volume ejected into a stiff aorta will elevate systolic and lower diastolic pressure. Thus, bradycardia often causes systolic hypertension, or makes it very resistant to therapy. Heart rate progressively slows throughout life and bradycardia is common in elderly patients. Bradycardia can be aggravated by underlying sick sinus syndrome and other conduction abnormalities or, more commonly, beta-blocker therapy. Beta-blockers, therefore, are not useful in the treatment of isolated systolic hypertension. Conversely, a dihydropyridine calcium antagonist, possibly in combination with an ACE inhibitor or an ARB, is prone to lower systolic pressure into, or at least close to, the target range. Of note, BP in elderly patients can be exquisitely sensitive to antihypertensive therapy; therefore, initiation of any drug should start at low doses and be uptitrated very gradually at an interval of 2–4 months. Low-dose diuretic therapy is often a helpful adjunct, although the propensity of diuretics to cause hyponatremia in the geriatric population, particularly in women, should be remembered.

## The "I want to do it the natural way" patient

Not uncommonly, the physician is challenged by a patient who insists on doing it his or her own "natural" way. Even though most physicians recognize that this endeavor will be futile, an enthusiastic patient should be encouraged to exercise regularly, lose weight and follow a healthy sodium-restricted diet. The only harm that can come from this is that BP remains elevated and the cardiovascular system of the patient continues to be exposed to a high pressure load. It is therefore important to monitor these patients carefully. In this context, the 24-hour ambulatory BP monitor is very useful and allows you to confront the patient with the before and after BP pattern. Very often, there is little difference between the two, and the evidence suffices to motivate the patient to start antihypertensive therapy. Home BP monitoring is less objective because patients have a tendency to cherry pick good BP readings, record these and then bring them to their physician. A good part of "white-coat" hypertension may be due to cherry picking of BP levels at home.

## The "nothing works/allergic to everything" patient

These patients are also called "heart sink" patients because the physician's heart sinks whenever they show up in the waiting room. What, perhaps, is most important with patients like this is to try to sort the wheat from the chaff. Thus, a very thorough, detailed history regarding previous medications, duration of use and reasons for discontinuation can often provide an astonishing insight. If a patient who is "allergic to everything" lists among these allergies a dry cough with certain drugs, or pedal edema with others, the physician has to take the reported adverse events more seriously and try to find a drug that the patient can tolerate. Commonly, the patient is willing to be rechallenged when the options are carefully explained. Using low-dose aspirin, and even iron supplements, can mitigate the cough seen with ACE inhibitors. Consider that some patients may be perfectly willing to continue with the ACE inhibitor, despite the persistence of a low-grade cough. Similarly, a patient who is "allergic" to dihydropyridine calcium antagonists because of pedal edema may be willing to be rechallenged when it is explained that, in combination with an ACE inhibitor or an ARB, the pedal edema is much less likely to occur. Gingival hyperplasia, which occurs occasionally with calcium antagonists, can be mitigated by concomitant therapy with an ACE inhibitor or an ARB, although it takes much longer for hyperplasia to regress than for pedal edema to subside. With a few exceptions, the adverse effects associated with most cardiovascular drugs occur within the first few days or weeks of therapy, although some (for instance, angioedema with ACE inhibitors) can occur after many months. Unfortunately, the patient who is "allergic to everything" tends to blame any symptom, from shin splints to female itch, on the antihypertensive drug, even if it occurs weeks or months after therapy is begun. Very often, this presents a high degree of underlying anxiety that taking any medication for a prolonged period of time is likely to have a negative impact on health ("this drug can destroy my kidneys"). As a consequence of this anxiety, many patients switch to "more natural" medicines that they find in health food stores. Although the concerns surrounding long-term safety of approved cardiovascular drugs have not been laid to rest, these drugs are still a lot safer than most concoctions sold in health food stores, where neither safety, nor efficacy, has ever been scrutinized.

Patients in whom "nothing works" should be told that all antihypertensive drugs lower BP but that this efficacy may vary from one patient to the other; one size does not fit all. The only drug class that has been shown, in some patients, to paradoxically elevate BP are the beta-blockers. The blockers of the RAS (ie, ARBs and ACE inhibitors) are less effective in patients who are on a high salt intake, in patients on NSAIDs or COX2 inhibitors, and also in black patients. However, despite lowering BP less well, these drugs still exert protection for the kidney, the heart, and the vascular tree. Very often, this pseudo-resistance can be abolished by the addition of a second drug, such as a diuretic or a calcium antagonist.

The "nothing works/allergic to everything" patients are often so convinced of their body being special, and their BP not responding to anything, that even the most sophisticated therapeutic efforts of the treating physician are counter-productive. In a situation like this (which needless to say is extremely frustrating for the physician), it may be helpful to go over the goals of antihypertensive therapy, not necessarily only to lower BP, but also to prevent heart attacks and strokes, the failure of which to treat would, very simply, increase the risk of these events ("We cannot prevent you from dying, but we can possibly prevent you from having a stroke"). In this context, it should be emphasized that many patients have high BP and live with it for years without ever having a heart attack or a stroke. Conversely, many patients with perfectly normal BP also suffer heart attacks and strokes. Therefore, antihypertensive treatment is not "mandatory" but, very simply, alters the risk/benefit ratio; it lowers the risk of some of the most devastating and dreaded diseases. By shifting the burden of decision making and evaluation of the risk/benefit ratio to the patient, often a different level of insight and compliance with antihypertensive drug therapy can be achieved.

In this process of coaching and hand-holding, it is important to remain vigilant with regard to any possible new, or yet unknown, adverse effects. Such adverse effects are more likely to occur in recently introduced drug classes than in diuretics that have been around for more than 40 years. However, only recently, it has been determined that long-term diuretic therapy is a low-grade risk for renal cell carcinoma. Also, it should be remembered that ACE inhibitors were used for quite some time before physicians realized that a dry cough, or angioedema, were adverse effects directly related to this drug class. Having exhausted the above suggestions, the best strategy may be to declare defeat and to admit, frankly, to the patient to be at the end of therapeutic wisdom. A referral to a specialist colleague may be helpful in this situation, as continuous frustration on either part, the patient's or the physician's, is not conducive to a good physician–patient relationship.

# Chapter 13

# Fashions and fads

## Sublingual nifedipine

Sublingual nifedipine is used worldwide to lower BP acutely in so-called hypertensive emergencies. Unfortunately, many patients who received sublingual nifedipine needed it about as much as a patient with high cholesterol would need a sublingual statin. Of note, there is good evidence that the sublingual application is of no added benefit because what gets into the blood stream is actually what is swallowed. Also, sublingual nifedipine lowers BP in a completely uncontrolled way, and such an abrupt BP drop has been associated with acute MI, stroke and death. Clearly, this is BP cosmetics and should be considered malpractice.

## Dual RAS blockade

### Blood pressure

Most BP studies showed a small additional drop in systolic and diastolic pressure when an ARB was added to an ACE inhibitor, and vice versa, regardless of the dose level of the first drug. A thorough systematic review and meta-analysis assessed 14 BP studies in hypertensive patients in which patients were evaluated by 24-hour ambulatory BP monitoring [91]. The authors found that the combination of an ACE inhibitor and an ARB reduced BP by an average of 4/3 mmHg when compared with monotherapy. The incremental fall in BP with dual RAS blockade compared with that seen with monotherapy is certainly only a fraction of what is commonly observed with the addition of either a thiazide or calcium antagonist.

### Albuminuria

So-called benefits of dual RAS blockade were reported in patients with albuminuria when compared with monotherapy with either an ARB or an ACE inhibitor [92]. In a meta-analysis of 49 studies involving over 6,000 patients, Kunz *et al.* [93] found "encouraging" evidence that dual RAS blockade reduced proteinuria by more than 20–25% when compared with either drug alone. The most recent landmark study, the ONTARGET study, is no exception in this regard [94]. The increase in albuminuria was reduced by a combination of telmisartan and ramipril when compared with monotherapy. However, the finding of significantly greater doubling of creatinine and dialysis in the combination arm, despite the lesser albuminuria, strongly argues against a nephroprotective effect of dual RAS inhibition.

These findings from the ONTARGET study clearly emphasize the fallacy of the surrogate end point (ie, the surrogate, albuminuria, moves in the "right" direction, whereas the real end point, doubling of creatinine and dialysis, moves in the opposite direction). This divergence between the real and surrogate end points should not be surprising in view of the experimental studies in sodium-depleted animals [95].

## Heart failure

The CHARM-Added (effects of candesartan in patients with chronic heart failure and reduced left-ventricular systolic function taking angiotensin-converting-enzyme inhibitors) trial reported some benefits when candesartan was added to an ACE inhibitor in patients with New York Heart Association functional class III to IV heart failure and a left ventricular ejection fraction of 40% or lower [96]. The addition of candesartan reduced all components of the primary outcome and the total number of hospital admissions for heart failure, but not all-cause mortality. A meta-analysis looking at all of the studies in aggregate, including the CHARM-Added trial, found no reduction in all-cause mortality but a 23% reduction in heart failure hospitalizations [97]. Of note, in the CHARM-Added trial, significantly more patients discontinued study medication in the combination arm because of an adverse event or abnormal laboratory values (increase in creatinine, hyperkalemia) in the combination therapy arm than in the placebo/ACE inhibitor arm. Indeed, a recent thorough meta-analysis looking at safety and tolerability of dual RAS blockade in over 18,000 patients with left ventricular dysfunction showed a significantly increased risk of adverse events, leading to discontinuation of dual RAS blockade compared with monotherapy [98]. Hypotension, a worsening of renal function, and hyperkalemia (ORs of 1.91, 2.12, and 4.17, respectively) were more common with combination therapy than with the ACE inhibitor alone. The authors concluded that this excess risk coupled with the lack of a consistent mortality benefit suggested that ARBs should not be added routinely to ACE inhibitors for left ventricular dysfunction [98].

## Direct renin inhibitors or aldosterone antagonists?

In a thorough prospective, randomized study of 599 patients, the mean urinary albumin to creatinine ratio was reduced by a further 20% following dual RAS blockade with aliskiren and losartan than with losartan alone, despite a very small difference in BP between the treatment groups [99]. The authors, apparently impressed by these results, enthusiastically concluded that "*aliskiren appears to have a renoprotective effect that is independent of its blood pressure-lowering effect*" [99]. However, given the surrogate end point failure in the ONTARGET study, the extrapolation from albuminuria to renal function is no longer acceptable. Clearly, to establish benefits, if any, of dual RAS blockade with direct renin inhibitors, ironclad outcome data on renal function will need to be provided. Indeed, such a study – the ALTITUDE study [51] – is currently in progress.

In contrast, in dual RAS blockade with aldosterone antagonists, such as spironolactone and eplerenone, both the surrogate end point and the real end point move in parallel. Thus, at least in heart failure, the benefits of adding spironolactone or eplerenone to either an ACE inhibitor or an ARB have been well documented.

In conclusion, the recent ONTARGET study data [94] have shattered the halo of dual RAS blockade not only for hypertension but also for nephroprotection. The meta-analysis of Lakhdar et al. [98] has cast doubts on the safety of dual RAS blockade in patients with left ventricular dysfunction. In retrospect, many enticing features of dual RAS blockade were based on surrogate end point findings and, therefore, may have represented more wishful thinking rather than solid science. This would indicate that the FDA's reluctance to accept albuminuria/proteinuria as a valid surrogate is well founded [100]. Leapfrogging of surrogate data can no longer substitute for patient exposure in clinical outcome studies [101]. Unless data emerge to the contrary, dual RAS blockade should be considered dead until further notice.

## Dual calcium channel blockade

Occasionally, the combination of a dihydropyridine and a nondihydropyridine calcium antagonist may be considered. There is some evidence of an additive effect of this combination and it seems, in general, to be well tolerated [102]. Pedal edema is not aggravated by the addition of a nondihydropyridine calcium antagonist to a dihydropyridine agent. The combination may be particularly useful in patients with renal failure and hyperkalemia in whom RAS blockade has become relatively contraindicated. However, it must be emphasized that there are only a very few studies in a small number of patients reporting antihypertensive efficacy. Thus, there is surrogate end point evidence only, and no data indicate that the combination reduces morbidity and mortality.

# References

1.    Vasan RS, Larson MG, Leip EP et al. Impact of high-normal blood pressure on the risk of cardiovascular disease. N Engl J Med 2001; 345:1291–1297.
2.    Chobanian AV, Bakris GL, Black HR, et al; Joint National Committee on Prevention, Detection, Evaluation, and Treatment of High Blood Pressure. National Heart, Lung, and Blood Institute; National High Blood Pressure Education Program Coordinating Committee. Seventh report of the Joint National Committee on Prevention, Detection, Evaluation, and Treatment of High Blood Pressure. Hypertension 2003; 42:1206–1252.
3.    Cushman WC, Evans GW, Byington RP, et al; for the ACCORD Study Group. Effects of intensive blood-pressure control in type 2 diabetes mellitus. N Engl J Med 2010; 362:1575–1585.
4.    Messerli FH, Mancia G, Conti CR, et al. Dogma disputed: can aggressively lowering blood pressure in hypertensive patients with coronary artery disease be dangerous? Ann Intern Med 2006; 144:884–893.
5.    Aksnes TA, Kjeldsen SE, Rostrup M, et al. Impact of new-onset diabetes mellitus on cardiac outcomes in the Valsartan Antihypertensive Long-term Use Evaluation (VALUE) trial population. Hypertension 2007; 50:467–473.
6.    LaRosa JC, Grundy SM, Waters DD, et al; Treating to New Targets (TNT) Investigators. Intensive lipid lowering with atorvastatin in patients with stable coronary disease. N Engl J Med 2005; 352:1425–1435.
7.    Yusuf S, Teo KK, Pogue J, et al; ONTARGET Investigators. Telmisartan, ramipril, or both in patients at high risk for vascular events. N Engl J Med 2008; 358:1547–1559.
8.    Whelton SP, Chin A, Xin X, et al. Effect of aerobic exercise on blood pressure: a meta-analysis of randomized, controlled trials. Ann Intern Med 2002; 136:493–503.
9.    Cutler JA, Follmann D, Allender PS. Randomized trials of sodium reduction: an overview. Am J Clin Nutr 1997; 65(Suppl):643S–651S.
10.   Xin X, He J, Frontini MG, et al. Effects of alcohol reduction on blood pressure: a meta-analysis of randomized controlled trials. Hypertension 2001; 38:1112–1117.
11 .  Whelton PK, He J. Potassium in preventing and treating high blood pressure. Semin Nephrol 1999; 19:494–499.
12.   Franse LV, Pahor M, Di Bari M, et al. Hypokalemia associated with diuretic use and cardiovascular events in the Systolic Hypertension in the Elderly Program. Hypertension 2000; 35:1025–1030.
13.   Appel LJ, Moore TJ, Obarzanek E, et al. A clinical trial of the effects of dietary patterns on blood pressure. DASH Collaborative Research Group. N Engl J Med 1997; 336:1117–1124.
14.   Sacks FM, Campos H. Dietary therapy in hypertension. N Engl J Med 2010; 362:2102–2112.
15.   Sjöström CD, Peltonen M, Sjöström L. Blood pressure and pulse pressure during long-term weight loss in the obese: the Swedish Obese Subjects (SOS) Intervention Study. Obes Res 2001; 9:188–195.
16.   Schmieder RE, Rockstroh JK, Messerli FH. Antihypertensive therapy. To stop or not to stop? JAMA 1991; 265:1566–1571.
17.   Messerli RH, Grossman E, Goldbourt U. Are beta-blockers efficacious as first-line therapy for hypertension in the elderly? A systematic review. JAMA 1998; 279:1903–1907.
18.   SHEP Cooperative Research Group. Prevention of stroke by antihypertensive drug treatment in older persons with isolated systolic hypertension. Final results of the Systolic Hypertension in the Elderly Program (SHEP). SHEP Cooperative Research Group. JAMA 1991; 265:3255–3264.

19. Antihypertensive and Lipid-Lowering Treatment to Prevent Heart Attack Trial Collaborative Research Group. Diuretic versus alpha-blocker as first-step antihypertensive therapy: final results from the Antihypertensive and Lipid-Lowering Treatment to Prevent Heart Attack Trial (ALLHAT). Hypertension 2003; 42:239–246.

20. Beckett NS, Peters R, Fletcher AE et al.; and the HYVET Study Group. Treatment of hypertension in patients 80 years of age or older. N Engl J Med 2008; 358:1887–1898.

21. PROGRESS Collaborative Group. Randomised trial of a perindopril-based blood-pressure-lowering regimen among 6105 individuals with previous stroke or transient ischaemic attack. Lancet 2001; 358:1033–1041.

22. Messerli FH, Verdecchia P, et al. Antihypertensive efficacy of hydrochlorothiazide as evaluated by ambulatory blood pressure monitoring: a meta-analysis of randomized trials. 2010; In Submission.

23. Messerli FH. Evolution of calcium antagonists: past, present, and future. Clin Cardiol 2003; 26(Suppl 2):II12–II16.

24. Conroy RM, Pyörälä K, Fitzgerald AP, et al; on behalf of the SCORE project group. Estimation of ten-year risk of fatal cardiovascular disease in Europe: the SCORE project . Eur Heart J 2003; 24:987–1003.

25. Messerli F, Williams B, Ritz E. Essential hypertension. Lancet 2007; 370:591–603.

26. Yusuf S, Wittes J, Friedman L. Overview of results of randomized clinical trials in heart disease. JAMA 1988; 260:2088–2093.

27. ACE Inhibitor Myocardial Infarction Collaborative Group. Indications for ACE inhibitors in the early treatment of acute myocardial infarction: systematic overview of individual data from 100 000 patients in randomized trials. Circulation 1998; 97:2202–2212.

28. Flather MD, Yusuf S, Kober L, et al. Long-term ACE-inhibitor therapy in patients with heart failure or left-ventricular dysfunction: a systematic overview of data from individual patients. ACE-Inhibitor Myocardial Infarction Collaborative Group. Lancet 2000; 355:1575–1581.

29. Abe M, Okada K, Matsumoto K. Clinical experience in treating hypertension with fixed-dose combination therapy: angiotensin II receptor blocker losartan plus hydrochlorothiazide. Expert Opin Drug Metab Toxicol 2009; 5:1285–1303.

30. Chrysant SG, Cohen M. Sustained blood pressure control with controlled-release isradipine (isradipine-CR). J Clin Pharmacol 1995; 35:239–243.

31. Wald DS, Law M, Morris JK, et al. Combination therapy versus monotherapy in reducing blood pressure: meta-analysis on 11,000 participants from 42 trials. Am J Med 2009; 122:290–300.

32. Julius S, Kjeldsen SE, Weber M, et al; VALUE trial group. Outcomes in hypertensive patients at high cardiovascular risk treated with regimens based on valsartan or amlodipine: the VALUE randomised trial. Lancet 2004; 363:2022–2031.

33. Lewington S, Clarke R, Qizilbash N, et al; Prospective Studies Collaboration. Age-specific relevance of usual blood pressure to vascular mortality: a meta-analysis of individual data for one million adults in 61 prospective studies. Lancet 2002; 360:1903–1913.

34. Julius S, Nesbitt SD, Egan BM, et al.; for the Trial of Preventing Hypertension (TROPHY) Study Investigators. Feasibility of treating prehypertension with an angiotensin-receptor blocker. N Engl J Med 2006; 354:1685–1697.

35. Messerli FH, Bangalore S, Julius S. Risk/benefit assessment of beta-blockers and diuretics precludes their use for first-line therapy in hypertension. Circulation 2008; 117:2706–2715.

36. O'Donnell M. A Sceptic's Medical Dictionary. London; BMJ Books; 1997.

37. Messerli FH, Sulicka J, Gryglewska B. Treatment of hypertension in the elderly. N Engl J Med 2008; 359:972–973; author reply 973–974.

38. Pitt D. ACE inhibitor co-therapy in patients with heart failure: rationale for the Randomized Aldactone Evaluation Study (RALES). Eur Heart J 1995; 16(Suppl N):107–110.

39.  The sixth Report of the Joint National Committee on Prevention, Detection, Evaluation, and Treatment of High Blood Pressure. Arch Intern Med 1997; 157:2413–2446.

40.  Medical Research Council trial of treatment of hypertension in older adults: principal results. MRC Working Party. BMJ 1992; 304:405–412.

41.  Kostis JB, Berge KG, Davis BR, et al. Effect of atenolol and reserpine on selected events in the systolic hypertension in the elderly program (SHEP). Am J Hypertens 1995; 8:1147–1153.

42.  Poole-Wilson PA, Swedberg K, Cleland JG, et al. Comparison of carvedilol and metoprolol on clinical outcomes in patients with chronic heart failure in the Carvedilol Or Metoprolol European Trial (COMET): randomised controlled trial. Lancet 2003; 362:7–13.

43.  The ALLHAT Officers and Co-ordinators for the ALLHAT Collaborative Group. Major outcomes in high-risk hypertensive patients randomized to angiotensin converting enzyme inhibitor or calcium channel blocker vs diuretic. The Antihypertensive and Lipid-Lowering Treatment to Prevent Heart Attack Trial (ALLHAT). JAMA 2002; 288:2981–2997.

44.  Effects of enalapril on mortality in severe congestive heart failure. Results of the Cooperative North Scandinavian Enalapril Survival Study (CONSENSUS). The CONSENSUS Trial Study Group. N Engl J Med 1987; 316:1429–1435.

45.  Cohn JN, Tognoni G; Valsartan Heart Failure Trial Investigators. A randomized trial of the angiotensin-receptor blocker valsartan in chronic heart failure. N Engl J Med 2001; 345:1667–1675.

46.  Weir RA, McMurray JJ, Puu M, et al; CHARM Investigators. Efficacy and tolerability of adding an angiotensin receptor blocker in patients with heart failure already receiving an angiotensin-converting inhibitor plus aldosterone antagonist, with or without a beta blocker. Findings from the Candesartan in Heart failure: Assessment of Reduction in Mortality and morbidity (CHARM)-Added trial. Eur J Heart Fail 2008; 10:157–163.

47.  Schmieder RE, Philipp T, Guerediaga J, et al. Long-term antihypertensive efficacyand safety of the oral direct renin inhibitor askiliren: a 12-month randomized, double-blind comparator trial with hydrochlorothiazide. Circulation 2009; 119:417–425.

48.  Schmieder RE, Philipp T, Guerediaga J, Gorostidi M, Keefe DL. Aliskiren-based therapy lowers blood pressure more effectively than hydrochlorothiazide-based therapy in obese patients with hypertension: sub-analyses of a 52-week, randomized, double-blind trial. J Hypertens. 2009; 27:1493–1501.

49.  Mogensen CE, Neldam S, Tikkanen I, et al. Randomised controlled trial of dual blockade of renin-angiotensin system in patients with hypertension, microalbuminuria, and non-insulin dependent diabetes: the candesartan and lisinopril microalbuminuria (CALM) study. BMJ 2000; 321:1440–1444.

50.  Oparil S, Yarows SA, Patel S, et al. Efficacy and safety of combined use of aliskiren and valsartan in patients with hypertension: a randomised, double-blind trial. Lancet 2007; 370:221–229.

51.  Parving HH, Brenner BM, McMurray JJ, et al. Aliskiren Trial in Type 2 Diabetes Using Cardio-Renal Endpoints (ALTITUDE): rationale and study design. Nephrol Dial Transplant 2009; 24:1663–1671.

52.  Opie LH, Messerli FH. Combination Drug Therapy for Hypertension. New York: Author's Publishing House, 1997.

53.  Pepine CJ, Handberg EM, Cooper-DeHoff RM, et al.; INVEST Investigators. A calcium antagonist vs a non-calcium antagonist hypertension treatment strategy for patients with coronary artery disease. The International Verapamil-Trandolapril Study (INVEST): a randomized controlled trial. JAMA 2003; 290:2805–2816.

54.  Dahlof B, Sever PS, Poulter NR, et al. Prevention of cardiovascular events with an antihypertensive regimen of amlodipine adding perindopril as required versus atenolol adding bendroflumethiazide as required, in the Anglo-Scandinavian Cardiac Outcomes Trial-Blood Pressure Lowering Arm (ASCOT-BPLA): a multicentre randomised controlled trial. Lancet 2005; 366:895–906.

55.  Messerli FH, Weir MR, Neutel JM. Combination therapy of amlodipine/benazepril versus monotherapy of amlodipine in a practice-based setting. Am J Hypertens 2002; 15:550–556.

56.  Messerli FH, Grossman E. Pedal edema – not all dihydropyridine calcium antagonists are created equal. Am J Hypertens 2002; 15:1019–1020.

57.  Weber MA, Bakris GL, Dahlof B, et al. Baseline characteristics in the Avoiding Cardiovascular events through Combination therapy in Patients Living with Systolic Hypertension (ACCOMPLISH) trial: a hypertensive population at high cardiovascular risk. Blood Press 2007; 16:13–19.

58.  Bangalore S, Kamalakkannan G, Parkar S, Messerli FH. Fixed-dose combinations improve medication compliance: a meta-analysis. Am J Med 2007; 120:713–719.

59.  Lewis PJ, Kohner EM, Petrie A, et al. Deterioration of glucose tolerance in hypertensive patients on prolonged diuretic treatment. Lancet 1976; 1:564–566.

60.  Murphy MB, Lewis PJ, Kohner E, Schumer B, Dollery CT. Glucose intolerance in hypertensive patients treated with diuretics; a 14-year follow-up. Lancet 1982; 2:1293–1295.

61.  Elliott WJ, Meyer PM. Incident diabetes in clinical trials of antihypertensive drugs: a network meta-analysis. Lancet 2007; 369:201–207.

62.  Lindholm LH, Persson M, Alaupovic P, et al. Metabolic outcome during 1 year in newly detected hypertensives: results of the Antihypertensive Treatment and Lipid Profile in a North of Sweden Efficacy Evaluation (ALPINE study). J Hypertens 2003; 21:1563–1574.

63.  Conn JW. Hypertension, the potassium ion and impaired carbohydrate tolerance. N Engl J Med 1965; 273:1135–1143.

64.  Helderman JH, Elahi D, Andersen DK, et al. Prevention of the glucose intolerance of thiazide diuretics by maintenance of body potassium. Diabetes 1983; 32:106–111.

65.  Verdecchia P, Reboldi G, Angeli F, et al. Adverse prognostic significance of new diabetes in treated hypertensive subjects. Hypertension 2004; 43:963–969.

66.  Alderman MH, Cohen H, Madhavan S. Diabetes and cardiovascular events in hypertensive patients. Hypertension 1999; 33:1130–1134.

67.  Elliott – reference unknown.

68.  Messerli FH, Bangalore S, Ruschitzka F. Angiotensin receptor blockers: baseline therapy in hypertension? Eur Heart J 2009; 30:2427–2430.

69.  Forette F, Seux ML, Staessen JA, et al. The prevention of dementia with antihypertensive treatment: new evidence from the Systolic Hypertension in Europe (Syst–Eur) study. Arch Intern Med 2002; 162:2046–2052.

70.  Lip GYH, Blann AD. Does hypertension confer a prothrombotic state? Virchow's triad revisited. Circulation 2000; 101:218–220.

71.  Taddei S, Virdis A, Ghiadoni L, Salvetti G, Salvetti A. Endothelial dysfunction in hypertension. J Nephrol 2000; 13:205–210.

72.  Spronk HM, Govers-Riemslag JW, ten Cate H. The blood coagulation system as a molecular machine. BioEssays 2003; 25:1220–1128.

73.  Boulanger CM. Secondary endothelial dysfunction: hypertension and heart failure. J Mol Cell Cardiol 1999; 31:39–49.

74.  Walters J, Skene D, Hampton SM, Ferns GA. Biological rhythms, endothelial health and cardiovascular disease. Med Sci Monit 2003; 9: RA1–8.

75.  Vapaatalo H, Mervaala E. Clinically important factors influencing endothelial function. Med Sci Monit 2001; 7:1075–185.

76.  Dielis AWJH, Smid M, Spronk HMH, et al. The prothrombotic paradox of hypertension: role of the renin-angiotensin and kallikrein-kinin systems. Hypertension 2005; 46:1236–1242.

77.  Naghavi M, Libby P, Falk E, et al. From vulnerable plaque to vulnerable patient: a call for new definitions and risk assessment strategies—part I. Circulation 2003; 108:1664–1672.

78. Ridderstråle W, Ulfhammer E, Jern S, Hrafnkelsdottir T. Impaired capacity for stimulated fibrinolysis in primary hypertension is restored by antihypertensive therapy. Hypertension 2006; 47:686–691.

79. Kalinowski L, Matys T, Chabielska E, Buczko W, Malinski T. Angiotensin II AT1 receptor antagonists inhibit platelet adhesion and aggregation by nitric oxide release. Hypertension 2002; 40:521–527.

80. Bakris GL, Weir MR, Secic M, et al. Differential effects of calcium antagonist subclasses on markers of nephropathy progression. Kidney Int 2004; 65:1991–2002.

81. Elliott WJ. Circadian variation in the timing of stroke onset: a meta-analysis. Stroke 1998; 29:992–996.

82. Kario K, Pickering TG, Hoshide S, et al. Morning blood pressure surge and hypertensive cerebrovascular disease: role of the alpha adrenergic sympathetic nervous system. Am J Hypertens 2004; 17:668–675.

83. Mancia G, Bombelli M, Facchetti R, et al. Long-term risk of sustained hypertension in white-coat or masked hypertension. Hypertension 2009; 54:226–232.

84. Messerli F, Makani H. Relentless progression toward sustained hypertension. Hypertension 2009; 254:217–218.

85. Brewster LM, van Montfrans GA, Kleijnen J. Systematic review: antihypertensive drug therapy in black patients. Ann Intern Med 2004; 141:614–627.

86. Douglas JG, Agodoa L.ACE inhibition is effective and renoprotective in hypertensive nephrosclerosis: the African American Study of Kidney Disease and Hypertension (AASK) trial. Kidney Int Suppl 2003; 83:S74–S76.

87. Dean DE, Schultz DL, Powers RH. Asphyxia due to angiotensin converting enzyme (ACE) inhibitor mediated angioedema of the tongue during the treatment of hypertensive heart disease. J Forensic Sci 2001; 46:1239–1243.

88. Llisteri JL, Vidal JVL, Aznar Vincente JA, et al. Sexual dysfunction in hypertensive patients treated with losartan. Am J Med Sci 2001; 321:336–341.

89. Kaplan NM. Hypertension Therapy Annual. London: Martin Dunitz, 2000.

90. Tordoir JH, Scheffers I, Schmidli J, et al. An implantable carotid sinus baroreflex activating system: surgical technique and short-term outcome from a multi-center feasibility trial for the treatment of resistant hypertension. Eur J Vasc Endovasc Surg 2007; 33:414–421.

91. Dulton TW, He FJ, MacGregor GA. Systematic review of combined angiotensin-converting enzyme inhibition and angiotensin receptor blockade in hypertension. Hypertension 2005; 45:880–886.

92. MacKinnon M, Shurraw S, Akbari A, et al. Combination therapy with an angiotensin receptor blocker and an ACE inhibitor in proteinuric renal disease: a systematic review of the efficacy and safety data. Am J Kidney Dis 2006; 48:8–20.

93. Kunz R, Friedrich C, Wolbers M, et al. Meta-analysis: effect of monotherapy and combination therapy with inhibitors of the renin angiotensin system on proteinuria in renal disease. Ann Intern Med 2008; 148:30–48.

94. Mann JF, Schmieder RE, McQueen M, et al. Renal outcomes with telmisartan, ramipril, or both, in people at high vascular risk (the ONTARGET study): a multicentre, randomised, double-blind, controlled trial. Lancet 2008; 372:547–553.

95. Griffiths CD, Morgan TO, Delbridge LM. Effects of combined administration of ACE inhibitor and angiotensin II receptor antagonist are prevented by a high NaCl intake. J Hypertens 2001; 19:2087–2095.

96. McMurray JJ, Ostergren J, Swedberg K, et al. Effects of candesartan in patients with chronic heart failure and reduced left-ventricular systolic function taking angiotensin-converting-enzyme inhibitors: the CHARM-Added trial. Lancet 2003;362:767–771.

97. Lee VC, Rhew DC, Dylan M, Badamgarav E, Braunstein GD, Weingarten SR. Meta-analysis: angiotensin-receptor blockers in chronic heart failure and high-risk acute myocardial infarction. Ann Intern Med 2004; 141:693–704.

98.	Lakhdar R, Al-Mallah MH, Lanfear DE. Safety and tolerability of angiotensin-converting enzyme inhibitor versus the combination of angiotensin-converting enzyme inhibitor and angiotensin receptor blocker in patients with left ventricular dysfunction: a systematic review and meta-analysis of randomized controlled trials. J Card Fail 2008; 14:181–188.

99.	Parving HH, Persson F, Lewis JB, et al; AVOID Study Investigators. Aliskiren combined with losartan in type 2 diabetes and nephropathy. N Engl J Med 2008; 358:2433–2446.

100.	Schlam E. NKF, FDA Host Conference to Assess Proteinuria as a Surrogate Outcome in CKD. New York, 2008. Available at: www.kidney.org/professionals/physicians/proteinuria.cfm. Accessed May 2011.

101.	Pfeffer MA, Sacks FM. Leapfrogging data: no shortcuts for safety or efficacy information. Circulation 2008; 118:2491–2494.

102.	Alviar, CL, DevarapallyS, Romero J, et al. Efficacy and safety of dual calcium channel blocker therapy for the treatment of hypertension: a meta-analysis. Presented at: American Society for Hypertension 25th Annual Scientific Meeting; May 1–4, 2010; New York, NY.